3000 800028 65631
St. Louis Community College

W9-DBK-309

WITHDRAWN

F V

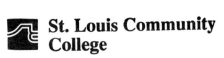 **St. Louis Community
College**

Forest Park
Florissant Valley
Meramec

Instructional Resources
St. Louis, Missouri

GAYLORD

SOCIAL PROBLEM SOLVING

The Guilford School Practitioner Series

EDITORS

STEPHEN N. ELLIOTT, Ph.D.
University of Wisconsin–Madison

JOSEPH C. WITT, Ph.D.
Louisiana State University, Baton Rouge

Recent Volumes

Social Problem Solving

INTERVENTIONS IN THE SCHOOLS

♦♦♦

Maurice J. Elias, Ph.D.
Steven E. Tobias, Psy.D.

♦

THE GUILFORD PRESS
New York   London

© 1996 The Guilford Press
A Division of Guilford Publications, Inc.
72 Spring Street, New York, NY 10012

All rights reserved

No part of this book may be reproduced, stored in a retrieval
system, or transmitted, in any form or by any means, electronic,
mechanical, photocopying, microfilming, recording, or otherwise,
without written permission from the Publisher.

Printed in the United States of America

This book is printed on acid-free paper.

Last digit is print number: 9 8 7 6 5 4 3 2 1

Library of Congress Cataloging-in-Publication Data

Elias, Maurice J.
    Social problem solving : interventions in the schools / Maurice J.
Elias, Steven E. Tobias.
        p.   cm. — (The Guilford school practitioners series)
    Includes bibliographical references and index.
    ISBN 1-57230-072-8
    1. Social skills—Study and teaching.   2. Social skills in
children—Study and teaching.   I. Tobias, Steven E.   II. Title.
III. Series.
HQ783.E425   1996
302'.14—dc20   95-53954
                                                                CIP

To my wife, Ellen,
and to Sara Elizabeth and Samara Alexandra,
as well as to my parents, Agnes and Sol,
and in-laws, Myra and Lou Rosen,
I (MJE) give my love;
my thanks for your forbearance, fortification,
invigoration, and inspiration;
and a briefly vacated space near the computer.

To my wife, Carol,
and to Meg and Gillian,
I (SET) express my gratitude
for your love, understanding, and support.
Although it always pains me to be away from you,
I thank you for allowing me the time
to devote to this and other projects
so that I may try to improve the lives of all children.

Preface

♦

For students to enter the community of responsible adults prepared for a diversity of social roles, they must possess critical-thinking and problem-solving skills, as well as interpersonal sensitivity. Their future success in citizenship, parenthood, family life, and the workplace will require them to find appropriate answers to numerous difficult questions, and it is up to the schools to help provide a foundation from which to answer them. Furthermore, there is no school without a moral or mandated imperative to prevent students' behavior problems, substance abuse, AIDS, and related difficulties. To these ends, innovative methods exist that can be of practical use to virtually all school practitioners.

The paths to violence, social withdrawal, disciplinary problems, and poor motivation can become set even by the end of the elementary school years, so early action is needed. For many children, this is a time of moving in positive and hopeful directions, or entering negative downward spirals. Indeed, the time to put a stop to the dynamics that lead to such problems as school disaffection and failure is during the elementary school and middle school years. This is equally true with regard to drug and alcohol use, smoking, sexual behavior, delinquency, school dropout, and, of course, HIV/AIDS.

There is a snowballing movement in America to provide children with the skills needed for the kind of clear thinking that leads to positive health behaviors, sound peer relationships, and the motivation to use school as a place of learning. These skills are the same ones that are needed to prevent substance abuse and other high-risk behaviors. We must prepare children to be able to respond thoughtfully in decision-making or problem-solving situations. Although these situations already occur as children proceed through their social and academic routines, children will face increasingly greater challenges as the years pass. The skills needed for children to handle these situations competently are referred to as *social problem-solving and decision-making skills.* These skills involve (1) a core set of thinking skills essential for successful decision making, such as the ability to understand signs of one's own and others' feelings, the ability to decide on one's goals, and the ability to think in terms of long- and short-term consequences as well as consequences both for oneself and others, (2) a set of "readiness" or learning-to-learn skills, which include the main areas of increasing self-control and building social skills for group participation and social awareness; and (3) explicit guidance in applying social decision-making skills in academic and interpersonal situations that occur throughout the school day.

Our point of view is that social problem-solving and everyday decision-making skills are essential to sound growth and development. Learning social problem solving and everyday decision making is a developmental right of all children, and systematic instruction in those skills—particularly beginning at the early grades—is of equal relevance to children's future in a social world as instruction in "traditional" academic skills. Indeed, we could argue that social problem-solving and decision-making skills are primary, without which success in social and vocational spheres is impossible. When children have difficulties that lead to a need for treatment in psychiatric clinics, mental health centers, adolescent treatment facilities, and the like, it usually is discovered that they have deficiencies in social problem-solving and everyday decision-making skills. Treatment often consists of providing them with those skills. But not all children get the help they need when they need it. Resources are scarce and access is not always equitable. And why must trouble be the signal to provide a basic and necessary learning experience? The harsh price of "starting too late" does not require elaboration to those who work with children and families.

A related aspect of our point of view—and something that is distinctive about social problem solving and decision making when compared to other approaches in the social and affective, critical thinking, and prevention domains—is the extent to which our instructional procedures and activities emphasize the application of skills and concepts learned in the classroom to a range of everyday academic and social contexts. We neither hope for transfer of learning, nor do we expect it. Rather, for the benefit of educators and other readers, the approach is deliberately structured to foster application of learning to real life.

The program presented in this book differs from other social skills and related programs in another way. This book was written to serve as a practical inservice training program with specific techniques and activities that can be used by any school staff member, from part-time lunch aide to school principal, without a major commitment of time, training, resources, or support staff. We wrote the book in this manner because we know the realities under which school personnel usually have to operate, that is, with little available time, training, resources, or support staff.

"FIG TESPN" is the centralizing concept of the program. It is an acronym for a set of social problem-solving and everyday decision-making steps (see Table 1.1 in Chapter 1) that are essential for success in school, with family, with friends, in the world of work, and in the exercise of the privileges and obligations of citizenship in a democracy. The steps themselves have much in common with those of other programs and many will be familiar to readers. We believe, however, that FIG TESPN is unique in that it provides continuity and consolidation of the process of learning and applying social problem solving and everyday decision making. Learning is then solidified through application of the process to a wide range of academic and social areas.

WHAT IS THE BACKGROUND OF THIS WORK?

The social problem-solving and decision-making approaches in this book provide those who work with children and adolescents with the tools to create "communities" that nurture both the human spirit and the intellect. They promote the critical thinking and the social and life skills needed to improve the ability of children to access and enact successfully a range of social roles.

The ideas and practices in this book flow from the work of the Improving Social Awareness–Social Problem Solving (ISA-SPS) Project, an ongoing, multiyear collaboration between school-based and agency-based professionals working from a social problem-solving and everyday decision-making model, and Psychological Enterprises, Incorporated, an innovative partnership linking social problem solving and everyday decision making to modern intervention technology. The areas of self-control, group participation and social awareness, and social–cognitive problem-solving and decision-making skills are key components of interventions reaching children at high, moderate, and low levels of risk, in both agency, clinical, and school contexts.

We are licensed clinical, school, and community psychologists who describe and illustrate applications of preventive and remediative programs based on social problem solving. Of all of our roles, we are most proud of being practitioners who put the techniques in this book to frequent use in applied settings. The interventions presented reflect the key elements underlying successful intervention design, using models recognized as outstanding by the U.S. Department of Education's Program Effectiveness Panel of the National Diffusion Network (NDN) and the National Educational Goals Panel, the National Mental Health Association, and the American Psychological Association. A spectrum of applications is featured, including state-of-the-art computer-based discipline enhancement and problem-solving procedures that can be used by school practitioners and in any school.

INTENDED USES OF THIS BOOK

The school practitioner of the 21st century will have to master instructional modalities and implementation technologies that are flexible, given the changing forms of school organization and classroom instruction. What will *not* change are basic principles of effective learning and the importance of certain key skills for everyday social, academic, familial, and vocational success: self-control, group participation and social awareness, effective communication, positive and persistent work habits, and skills for solving everyday social problems and making academic and personal decisions and choices. Nor will there be any changes in the importance of building human relationships as a critical context for any learning activity.

Certain units of intervention technology and instructional delivery also will be stable during this time. These include the use of facilitative questioning/dialoging to promote reflective thinking and representational competence; the synergistic effects of carefully designed multimedia formats; instructional units that simultaneously build children's confidence, competence, and chances to practice and use what they are learning successfully (what we call the "3 C's"); small group instruction; principles of engaging learning; and consultation far more than direct modalities of intervention.

With these tools in hand, with ways to link them to the enduring skill areas, and with specific examples of how interventions have been fit into a range of different school routines and contexts, the school practitioner is ready for whatever specific intervention opportunities might come along. Our book is organized to reflect this perspective.

An important basis of this book is that, over the next two decades, school practice in fields such as school psychology, social work, guidance, learning disabilities, health education, and special education will vary and look different in amount and nature. There will continue to be inconsistencies, both within and across school districts, in degrees of collaboration and institutional support for the work of school psychology. Relatedly, education reform will bring changes, as will the growing movement toward inclusion. Amidst this background of flux and uncertainty, we have chosen to focus on enduring aspects of social competence and prevention theory, research, and practice; by so doing, we hope to empower current and future school practitioners to serve children effectively in the variety of organizational contexts in which they might find themselves.

WHERE HAS THIS APPROACH ACTUALLY WORKED?

Our book has been informed by years of collaborative field research and development with teachers, administrators, and parents, most prominently through the ISA-SPS Project of Rutgers University and the University of Medicine and Dentistry of New Jersey–Community Mental Health Center (UMDNJ-CMHC) at Piscataway. The ISA-SPS Project began in 1979 with local school district funds in Middlesex Borough, New Jersey, and has extended over time with research and development funds from the National Institute of Mental Health, the William T. Grant Foundation, the Schumann Fund for New Jersey, and service funds from county and state sources. The ISA-SPS Project has conducted summer institutes and year-round staff development programs since 1983. Classroom-based materials have been found to satisfy elements of family life education and health education requirements, and have been designated by the New Jersey Department of Education as a model for substance abuse prevention in the elementary grades. The National Association of Private Schools for Exceptional Children has featured social problem solving as a model program for special education. Materials for parents have received recognition by the American Psychological Association for Excellence in Psychology in the Media, and in 1988 the ISA-SPS Project received the Lela Rowland Prevention Award from the National Mental Health Association as the outstanding prevention program in the country. In 1989, the ISA-SPS Project's elementary-level curriculum was approved by the Program Effectiveness Panel of the U.S. Department of Education's NDN, and also received Developer/Demonstrator funding from the NDN for national dissemination as a federally validated program. In 1994, the National Education Goals Panel designated this work as an exemplary model for Goal 7: Safe, Drug-Free Schools and Disciplined Environments Conducive to Learning.

Now, the approach is supported by service delivery from the UMDNJ-CMHC at Piscataway's Social Problem Solving Unit, by continuing education provided through the Center for Applied Psychology at Rutgers University, and through Psychological Enterprises, Incorporated. The base of the Project's continuing research and development activities is in New Jersey, where districts of all kinds—large and small, urban and rural—and communities of all socioeconomic levels are working with social problem solving. In addition, persons from schools in New York, Oregon, Massachusetts, Washington, Illinois, Ohio, Maryland, Florida, Vir-

ginia, Pennsylvania, Michigan, Canada, Israel, and England have successfully carried out ISA-SPS programs. Throughout the Project's research
and development efforts, the active collaboration of school personnel at
all levels has helped our approach to be relevant, realistic, enjoyable, and
capable of fitting into a variety of niches in the educational routine.

Most specifically, the FIG TESPN model presented in this book is
teacher and school professional tested. It is conveyed in this book through
instructional and intervention parameters and specific examples of a
school-based approach to providing children with a solid foundation of social problem-solving and everyday decision-making skills for use at all
grade levels and with diverse student populations. The techniques and activities discussed in this book are designed to become infused into the daily practice of teachers and the daily routines of all schools. Initially, some
additional time must be devoted to implementing the activities in this
book. This should be viewed as an investment that will come to fruition in
part through a more orderly and efficient classroom and more thoughtful
learners. Larger benefits will appear as increases in social competence,
positive character, and achievement on the part of the students—hall-
marks of better preparation of students for the responsibilities of being
citizens and leaders in a democracy.

Acknowledgments

♦

Our work represents the result of many years of collaboration with school professionals of all disciplines: teachers, school psychologists, social workers, guidance counselors, learning disabilities specialists, school nurses and other health educators, speech correctionists, principals, vice-principals, special educators, school librarians, lunch aides, and bus drivers all come quickly to mind. Our collaborators also have included clinicians, parents, and, perhaps most of all, the children themselves.

Indeed, no one has been spared from our involvement, and no one has spared us from their feedback, comments, and suggestions. As our work has evolved over the past decade, we have incorporated many of those ideas. They have served to enrich, invigorate, and transform the work over time. Those of you who have worked with other social problem-solving approaches, interpersonal cognitive problem solving, social skills training, or interventions with similar names and backgrounds will find familiar things in this book. But we guarantee that you also will find innovation, as a result of what we have been able to capture and share from the contexts of practice.

We have many debts of gratitude, but we will limit ourselves to those that are most important. First of all, our closest colleague, Dr. Brian Friedlander, has been a wonderful collaborator and friend, a high-tech innovator, and patient practitioner of social problem solving. We have learned a lot from him. Second, we salute the continued hard work of the staff of the Social Problem Solving Unit of the University of Medicine and Dentistry–Community Mental Health Center at Piscataway, New Jersey, a service unit that exists for the purpose of carrying our school-based social problem solving interventions and has been doing so for a number of years. Third, we are grateful for the continuous infusion of talent, energy, and enthusiasm from undergraduates of Rutgers University and students of Rutgers' graduate programs in psychology, social work, and the Graduate School of Applied and Professional Psychology. Where would we be without you? And we must give great thanks to Sharon Panulla, Senior Editor at The Guilford Press, whose belief in and enthusiasm for this project rescued it when it seemed as if it was not destined to come to fruition. Besides being wonderfully knowledgeable, Sharon is a marvelous source of support and facilitative encouragement (i.e., she knows the difference between a nudge and a nag).

Last, and most important, we want to thank our families, whose patience while we worked on this book (and all the school-based intervention that is the source of this book) is nothing less than remarkable. We are fortunate indeed to always (and still!) have you to come home to, to lean on, to inspire us, and to make sure we don't get too carried away with projects like this.

Contents

♦

SOCIAL PROBLEM SOLVING

CHAPTER 1

♦♦♦

The Central Role of Social Problem Solving and Everyday Decision Making

♦

Inclusion. Violence. Alcohol and Other Drug Use.
Behavior Problems. Conflict Resolution. Peer Mediation.
Cultural Conflict. Community Service. Parent Involvement.
Character Development. School Discipline.

These are some of the issues that have joined the "three R's" as concerns of those who work in the schools, or depend on the schools to prepare children for adult roles. No matter how hard we wish or how deep we try to bury our heads in the sand, these concerns are not going away. They are reflected in the seventh National Education Goal, as formulated in the *Goals 2000* legislation passed in 1994: "By the year 2000, every school in the United States will be free of drugs, violence, and the unauthorized presence of firearms and alcohol and will offer a disciplined environment conducive to learning" (National Education Goals Panel, 1994, p. 11); further, Goals 3 and 5 speak to the importance of developing the skills needed for responsible citizenship and participation in a global economy. It would not be a radical vision to maintain that, in the 21st century, students will be considered "educated" to the extent to which they can make informed, responsible decisions that promote their own well-being and contribute to the well-being of others.

Educators and parents, in preparing the next generations of students for their roles as responsible citizens, must strengthen children's ability to think clearly, carefully, and sensitively, particularly when under stress. We have no illusions about the challenges involved in accomplishing this task. Too often, constructive efforts to help children are overmatched by media shallowness, negative peer pressure, perceived attractive alternatives to hard work, household tensions and disruptions of all kinds, and a sense of uprootedness caused by social mobility. Lacking stable attachments to provide a sense of security and positive guidance, many children find their values and goals influenced by media and peer portrayals of "the good life" and how to "make it to the top." Amidst these many competing pressures, school professionals struggle to find a focus, a meaningful way to engage children in building the reasoning skills that research has shown are necessary for a healthy future.

The kind of future we must envision is a multicultural one, accepting of diversity and focusing on strengths. As reflected in the work of Howard Gardner in the area of multiple intelligences, this means that we must open ourselves to all aspects of competence, including the verbal–linguistic and logical–mathematical, but also the kinesthetic, the spatial and artistic, and the musical. And Gardner points out two other forms of intelligence vital to healthy functioning: the interpersonal and intrapersonal (Armstrong, 1994; Gardner, 1993). The latter two, which are common denominators across all ethnic, racial, and cultural boundaries, represent the focus of the work to be described here.

In a related way, the National Professional School Health Organizations (1984) have defined "health" as encompassing basic academic competencies, psychological and physical well-being, vocational competencies, positive interpersonal skills and relationships, a sense of linkage with and responsibility to one's community, and an orientation toward law-abiding behavior. In each of these areas, the capacity to make informed decisions is essential for positive outcomes to be obtained (Elias, 1990). Fortunately, decision-making approaches can be implemented in ways that do not overload the curriculum (D. Johnson & Johnson, 1990; King, 1986; Kolbe, 1985; London, 1987). By so doing, school practitioners can foster a systematic emphasis on social problem solving and decision making as a core set of skills that underlie competent performance in many specific academic and interpersonal domains.

THE PERVASIVENESS OF SOCIAL PROBLEM SOLVING

Consider how often children, parents, and educators are placed in situations that require them to make important choices. Choices begin when the alarm clock rings, continue throughout the morning routine, and accompany individuals during school, work, household tasks, and interactions with others. Consider some of the situations many children face on a daily basis that require thoughtful problem solving and effective decision making:

- Should I work hard or not?
- Should I become involved in religion or not?
- Should I use drugs, alcohol, or tobacco or not?
- Should I risk pregnancy or not?
- Should I vandalize or not?
- Should I drop out or not?
- Should I try suicide or not?
- Should I follow my friends' advice or not?
- Should I respect my parents or teachers or not?

Children's pathways into adulthood in a democratic society are bound to their ability to exercise critical judgment and make decisions regardless of their innate ability, environmental opportunity, background circumstances, or cultural heritage. Their decisions reflect their personal identity and, collectively, shape our national character. Will they be oriented to contribute or consume? To create or to accept? To care or to stand by? To lead responsibly or to follow uncritically? Even simpler everyday decisions—what to wear, where to sit, what to eat—are linked to the more critical decisions mentioned above by a common set of skills that influence the choices that are made.

The central role of social problem solving and decision making in education has both an intellectual and an interpersonal basis. The former stems from recent work suggesting that children (and adults) are most likely to show the extent of their abilities in contexts that they value (Raven, 1987). Because the social context is so salient for most children—particularly children traditionally seen as "at risk"—instruction in social problem solving is likely to engage their abilities and serve as a force for specific and general cognitive, affective, and social growth. Rather than build on areas of weakness or disinterest, social problem solving focuses on areas of potential strength and high salience (e.g., even for a school phobic or shy child, social situations are highly salient). This, in turn, facilitates children's continued engagement with school. The Association for Supervision and Curriculum Development has indicated that decision-making skills are essential for success as workers and as people in our society, and that the teaching of these skills early in life serves to prevent the onset of problem behaviors such as substance abuse (Benard, Fafoglia, & Perone, 1987; Wales, Nardi, & Stager, 1986). To the extent that children are members of racial and ethnic minority groups, it becomes imperative that they possess the skills to analyze the often complex or ambiguous situations they are in, the feelings they are having, the choices available to them, and the implications of those choices (Elias, Hancock, Gager, & Chung, 1993; Gibbs, 1989; Rosado, 1986).

The interpersonal basis is summarized well by London (1987):

> The job of the schools is to make children competent intellectually . . . and decent interpersonally. They [children] probably cannot achieve these ends without a sense of altruism or achievement or integrity or self-control or self-esteem. They certainly cannot succeed if they are drunk, drugged, depressed, or anxious; if they are parents before they can be breadwinners; or if they must abandon school to escape brutality, neglect, or despair at home. (pp. 670–671)

EIGHT PRIMARY PROBLEM-SOLVING SKILL AREAS

Although there are many skills that clearly are necessary for social decision making, our research and development team has synthesized eight primary skill areas from traditions in education, psychology, and philosophy. These eight areas are presented in Table 1.1. (Also presented in Table 1.1 is an instructional version of these areas, heuristically labeled as "FIG TESPN"; this version will be discussed further in Chapter 4.) Research

TABLE 1.1. A Social Problem-Solving and Decision-Making Strategy: Eight Skill Areas

When children and adults are using their social problem-solving skills, they are doing the following:
1. Noticing signs of feelings.
2. Identifying issues or problems.
3. Determining and selecting goals.
4. Generating alternative solutions.
5. Envisioning possible consequences.
6. Selecting their best solution.
7. Planning and making a final check for obstacles.
8. Noticing what happened and using the information for future decision making and problem solving.

An instructional version of the social decision-making and problem-solving skills, given the acronym "FIG TESPN":
1. Feelings cue me to problem solve.
2. I have a problem.
3. Goals give me a guide.
4. Think of many possible things to do.
5. Envision end results (outcomes) for each option.
6. Select my best solution.
7. Plan the procedure, anticipate pitfalls (roadblocks), practice, and pursue it.
8. Notice what happened and now what?

has shown that deficiencies in these skill areas are a common denominator among children and adolescents who experience a variety of problems, including academic failure and dropout, substance abuse, antisocial behavior, teenage pregnancy, and social rejection (Asarnow, Carlson, & Guthrie, 1987; Benard et al., 1987; Botvin, 1985; Elias et al., 1986; Flaherty, Mracek, Olsen, & Wilcove, 1983; Freedman, Donahoe, Rosenthal, Schlundt, & McFall, 1978; Kazdin & Associates, 1987; King, 1986).

Further, these skills appear to be cross-culturally relevant, in that they are salient to everyday interpersonal functioning and the instructional methods used to convey the skills are related to those fostering multicultural learning and learning involving various learning style preferences and modalities (Brendtro, Brokenleg, & Van Bockern, 1991; Carnine, 1994; Jones, 1991; McCarthy, 1990; Shinn & McConnell, 1994).

To highlight the salience of these skill areas for effectiveness in school, peer, and home interactions, each area and its corresponding instructional step are described below.

1. *Noticing signs of feelings/Feelings cue me to problem solve.* There are two aspects of this skill: signs of different feelings in *oneself*, and signs in *others*. When children have decisions to make, problems to solve, or otherwise feel under stress, their first reaction is likely to be *emotional*, rather than intellectual. This is especially true in children below high school age. They may try to beguile the adults around them with their sophisticated language and cerebral airs, but we should not be taken in. Just try to remember your own years prior to (or even during) high school. Emotions are at the forefront.

Sometimes students are confused by their emotions. This can lead to panic, a fight or flight reaction, or to their giving up on what they were trying to accomplish. Therefore, students (and adults) are taught their Feelings Fingerprints (Elias & Clabby, 1989)—the unique way in which their bodies signal them that they are in distress. For some, the signal is sweaty palms; for others, a stomach ache; many experience headaches of various kinds, and some have backaches, rashes, stiff necks, dry mouths—the list can go on and on. By teaching students their Feelings Fingerprints and labeling the Fingerprints publicly, one helps them to differentiate difficult, unarticulated feelings. This allows feelings to be put into words and serves as a "cue" for students to use their other cognitive decision-making skills.

Awareness of feelings in others also serves as a powerful cue that one might have a problem to think about. However, to the extent to which students do not attend to signs of feelings in others, misinterpret them, or have a limited perspective from which to understand those signs, they may arrive at decisions and take actions based on faulty premises. For example, young children tend to see the world in terms of sad, mad, and glad. As they grow, their perspective on the world extends to other feelings, such as pride, worry, calmness, and disappointment. Children with emotional disturbances, however, are less likely to show progress in their ability to look for and label signs of feelings. For them to become effective social decision makers, it is necessary to expand their feelings vocabularies (Elias & Clabby, 1989).

Consider a special education student who is mainstreamed. More generally, think about a child who is left out of groups that he or she wants to belong to. This is a very critical situation that affects many children. They want to join the group, but either they are not asked or they have been rejected. Perhaps they have developed a reputation so that nobody ever asks them to join in. Interestingly, as adults, we first learn about the problem through signs of different feelings expressed by the student. Think about a student that you know who has been left out. Think about a time when you have been left out. What kinds of feelings have you experienced? Sadness, hurt, anger, frustration, confusion, and embarrassment all come to mind; it is painful to always be standing on the side by yourself, with everybody knowing it. If we teach students their Feelings Fingerprints and labels for a range of feelings, we give them ways to notice and describe what they are experiencing. Then, rather than reacting with fight, flight, or just by standing there and being overwhelmed by one's feelings, a student can learn to take constructive action.

We focus students on their feelings by asking, "How are you feeling now? How did you feel when you went up to the group and they said no (or, when you found out you were left out)? How were the others in the group feeling? What did you see or hear that helped you know how they were feeling?"

2. *Identifying the issues or problems/I have a problem.* Stressful or upset or uncomfortable feelings are usually a sign that one has a decision to make or a problem to resolve. By helping students move from their stress to identifying the issue or problem, we enable them to use their thinking skills. It is as if they move from their heart to their head. We encourage them to put the problem into words: "Tell yourself what the problem is. When else have you felt this way? What was happening? Try to say, 'I feel _____ because. . .'; or 'When _____ happens, I feel _____.'" These questions give a focus to our feelings and our decision-making efforts and also serve to identify similar "trigger" situations that have led to similar feelings in the past. If we take the example of the rejected student, we might learn that the student is feeling anger and frustration. So we ask the student to put the problem into words. How might you put this child's problem into words?: "I feel angry because I would like

to be part of the group, but I can't"; "When they say no to me and act mean to me, I feel frustrated."

3. *Determining and selecting goals / Goals give me a guide.* Deciding on one's goal is a necessary step in decision making and problem solving of any kind. Would we drive a car without knowing our destination? How much do we enjoy or benefit from meetings when the purposes are vague? Can you tell the difference between a school—or a classroom—with clear goals and one without them? Students growing up in families with little supervision, conflicting supervision from divorced parents, or mixed priorities between home and school inevitably feel stress due to unclear goals. Sometimes this leads to inactivity, incomplete activity along a number of fronts, or misdirected activity. Peer pressure can be thought of as relating to not knowing one's goals, or, as we say to students, "following others' goals for you."

The area of smoking in middle school students offers a clear example. Students most often smoke because they think their peers smoke and that their peers will be pleased if they smoke also. But children often overestimate the number of classmates who smoke and, when asked about smoking in one-on-one discussions, acknowledge that smoking really is not their goal.

We help children focus on their goals by reversing the problem statements they make and by asking, "What do you want to have happen? How do you want things to end up?" We encourage them to visualize (picture, imagine, draw in their minds, describe in words, envision, etc.) what they would like to have happen, and to reflect on how their actions will help or not help their goals to be reached.

4. *Generating alternative solutions / Think of many possible things to do.* This is a familiar concept, often referred to as "brainstorming," or the nonevaluative generation of as many solutions, options, or choices as possible. When one thinks of one's students, from preschool through high school, one is aware that some are more flexible than others. This applies to a number of areas, such as in overcoming roadblocks in math, doing experiments or creative writing, and relating to peers and authority figures. Flexible thinking is a learned skill. It begins by creating an attitude that encourages children to think that there often is more than one reasonable way to solve a problem, cope with a difficulty, or reach one's goal. By thinking of different options before acting, children are more likely to have better ideas, less likely to act impulsively, and unlikely to be passive and "stuck" when faced with a problem or decision.

Brainstorming is encouraged when we ask children to *think of all the things that might happen next*, whether in response to a section of a book the class is reading, a newspaper article or other current events story, a discipline problem the whole class is having, or when a student begins to think about options after high school.

5. *Envisioning possible consequences / Envision end results (outcomes) for each option.* Ask some students, "When I ask you to *think* about something you are going to do, what do you do?" Ask others, "When I ask you to *think* about what might happen before you do it, what do you do?" Finally, ask yourself what you do when you *think* about the consequences of something you might do. There is a tendency to ask students to "think" about consequences, but developmental research suggests it would be more effective to ask children to *envision* what might happen next because doing so stimulates and capitalizes on their representational skills (Copple, Sigel, & Saunders, 1979). In our work, especially around application of social problem solving to health promotion and to substance abuse prevention, we find that visualization is the best language for thinking about consequences. Students "think" about short- and long-term consequences, consequences for themselves and others, and alternative consequences more easily if we ask them to picture, imagine, describe, walk us through, make a visual video of, put on the mental monitor what might happen. Having a picture in mind to carry around helps extend consequential thinking and makes it more likely that when children are away from kindly adult influences, they will keep realistic, sensible outcomes of their actions in mind.

6. *Selecting their best solution / Select my best solution.* This deceptively simple skill has several key components. Phrased as it is, it emphasizes that the individual takes *responsibility* for actively selecting what to do (or not do). It also clarifies that the reference point for selecting an action is one's goal, plus avoiding harm to oneself or others. We encourage this skill by asking, "Which of these ideas do you think will help you reach your goal (without harming you or anyone else)?"

7. *Planning and making a final check for obstacles / Plan the procedure, anticipate pitfalls (roadblocks), practice, and pursue it.* Planning skills are being viewed more and more as among the key factors that protect children from harm due to difficult life circumstance (Rutter, 1987). Planning skills refer to the "who, what, when, where, how, with whom, and to whom" considerations that accompany making one's good ideas work. Indeed, we can think of many talented friends, colleagues, and relatives whose good ideas run aground for lack of thinking through and following through on the detailed steps necessary to make sure things happen as they should. There are reasons why teachers have plan books and use lesson *plans*, and why special education is organized around individualized education programs

and instructional guides. Well, the same reasons apply to everyday decision making and social problem solving! And because lessons do not always go as planned, we emphasize the idea of *make a final check for obstacles*. Put simply, "What could happen so that your plan might not work out?" Good planners *anticipate roadblocks*. They look ahead before they start and use this knowledge to bolster their plans, or perhaps just to be more "ready" to deal with resistance. Envision the students you work with. You will see that some handle frustration better than others; some always have that extra pen or pencil, or extra paper. Some students are very set in their ways and when things do not work out as planned, they seem to "fall apart." What you are describing are examples of children who vary in a learned skill area—the ability to plan and to anticipate and plan for obstacles.

We encourage skill development in students by asking them first asking them a lot of "who, what, when"-type questions once they have selected their best solutions, to help them have a more detailed image of what it is they will actually need to do. Sometimes, at this stage of social problem solving, it becomes clear that one's best solution is not feasible. If this seems true, it is time to go back to earlier steps, review one's other alternatives, and perhaps even reconsider one's goal. Once a student seems to have a plan, we will ask, "What might happen to keep your plan from working?" Sometimes, if we think there is an obstacle that students are overlooking, we might say, "What if you go up to Mrs. Rollins and she seems very, very busy?" or "What if you ask Mr. Heisler and he says he really can't talk to you right now?" It is our responsibility as adults to help children learn that the environment will not always be receptive to them, even if they have done an excellent job of social problem solving.

In our work with at-risk and special education students, we have been reminded over and over again of how fragile their sense of trust and security often is. When they finally agree to work with you, to work on social problem solving, to think through problems and choices and practice their plans, they are hurt tremendously when they try their best and the world rebuffs them. What we have found, however, is that by anticipating obstacles and roadblocks with them (e.g., "What if Ms. M. is having a bad day and won't respond nicely to you or even see you?"), they can be fortified by knowing they did their best, that their work and planning was not for nothing, and that they can still have trust and confidence in the adults who taught them social problem solving—as well as in themselves. We are trying to insulate them against what they otherwise might see as failure. (We have learned much about the difficulty special education and at-risk children encounter when trying to change and improve because of the interplay of their own negative expectancies and the fact that a human environment offers many chances for rebuffs. The focus on obstacles has been a potent antidote to negativity and a valuable aid to positive motivation and self-confidence.)

8. *Noticing what happened and using the information for future decision making and problem solving/Notice what happened and now what?* Turn your thoughts to recent conferences you have had with parents. It is likely that you have heard yourself or the parents say something like, "Jackie does the same things over and over again. It never works out. Doesn't Jackie ever learn?" or "Carmen repeats the same mistakes all the time. Doesn't Carmen remember what happened the other times?" The answer to these questions often is, "No." These children lack the *skill* of using the past to inform the future. They do not know how to recall their past experiences and see how those experiences can apply to what is happening now or to what might happen next. Jackie and Carmen may be in kindergarten, sixth grade, or juniors in high school. If they are going to function well in the adult world, they need help with this skill. When students learn to "try it and rethink it," they are learning that decision making and problem solving are *processes*. Our message is basic but important in a world of instant gratification: "Go try it. Then, let's talk about what happened. Let's see what we can learn from it. If it doesn't work quite right, let's take a closer look at what happened and figure out what to do next." We hope to spark a spirit of experimentation, a willingness to work toward a desired goal, to think about the past and use it in the future, and to inspire self-confidence—"YOU CAN DO IT!"

INCLUSION: WHERE SOCIAL PROBLEM-SOLVING SKILLS ARE NEEDED BY ALL

These skills, we believe, also are fundamental to the success of what is referred to as "inclusion." In our view, inclusion requires the establishment of common ground between all students, and the creation of an environment where all students feel that they belong and are encouraged to learn at their highest level (Schrag & Burnette, 1994). In order for inclusion to work, classes that include students with disabilities must focus on the issues of self-worth, acceptance, respect for others, friendship, and everyday problem solving and conflict resolution (Stainback, Stainback, East, & Sapon-Shevin, 1994).

In line with this focus, a principal goal of inclusion is to enhance students' social competence and peer relationships and to change the attitudes of teachers and students without disabilities so that they better understand and are more accepting of others' differences (Fuchs & Fuchs, 1994). As Gresham (1982) points out, research has not supported the assumption that mainstreamed handicapped students will learn appropriate social behavior simply from interacting with nonclassified peers. In fact, research indicates that mainstreamed students, by and large, have low levels of social interaction in regular education settings. Students with handicaps may be identified as "different" on the basis of their behavior even before they are formally classified or segregated into special education programs (Braaten, Kauffman, Braaten, Posgrove, & Nelson, 1988). These students are often treated with derision by their nonclassified peers, partly as a result of their deficits in social competence (Gartner & Lipsky, 1987). Research by Fox (1989) examined peer rejection among fourth, fifth, and sixth grade students classified as having learning disabilities. Mainstreaming was found to increase the risk of social rejection.

Thus, assuming that mainstreamed students will simply "pick up" proper social behavior from contact with nonclassified peers is insufficient to ensure social success. Active measures must be taken in the direct training of social skills.

However, focusing solely on the social skills deficits of classified students is only half the issue. Classified students are often met by stereotypes, preconceptions, and antagonistic and rejecting behavior on the part of their nonclassified peers (Gresham, 1984). Blaming this on the deficits of the classified students amounts, in effect, to "blaming the victim." In this case, nonclassified students are showing a marked lack of self-control, empathy, and general prosocial behavior. As such, it is apparent that focusing attention on the skills deficits of students with mild disorders does not go far enough.

These issues form the rationale for an inclusive group intervention that focuses on all three of Fuchs and Fuchs' (1994) goals for inclusion. Direct efforts must be made at improving social skills for *all* students through curriculum-based lessons in social skills and social-cognitive problem solving. Second, by bringing classified and nonclassified children together in a structured group setting, and by working toward increased interpersonal awareness and empathy, an effective program aims at unraveling negative stereotypes between these two groups. The third area indicates the need to provide social cohesion and a context for friendships to develop.

Finally, there are studies that indicate that an inclusion strategy is most effective when combined with a focus on social skills training, fostering of interpersonal relationships and use of cooperative learning within classrooms, and ongoing teacher efforts to build students' critical thinking and problem-solving skills (Fox, 1989; Hawkins, Doueck, & Lishner, 1988; Scruggs, Mastropieri, & Sullivan, 1994). Moreover, there is little evidence that simple physical inclusion, without psychological inclusion, will benefit mildly handicapped learners (Stainback et al., 1994). Thus, the intervention strategy of choice for this population is one that focuses on both the skills of the children and on their interpersonal learning environments. The following sections in this chapter provide an introduction to a specific social problem-solving program that is of particular promise for comprehensive, long-term effectiveness with mildly handicapped students.

Reading this no doubt has triggered many images and associations. Perhaps you see yourself carrying out some or many of these ideas already. Perhaps you see how relevant they are to your own personal decision making and problem solving and how the process of social problem solving can be useful to you personally and professionally (cf. "Decision Making for Me" in Clabby & Elias, 1986). Most likely, you have questions about how this is put into practice in the schools. While the rest of the book will focus on specific examples, some of the basic questions asked most often about social problem solving will be addressed next.

COMMONLY ASKED QUESTIONS ABOUT SOCIAL PROBLEM SOLVING

Having provided an introduction to social problem solving and some of its many applications, we recognize that we have raised as many questions as we have answered. Therefore, before adding more information, we thought we would address those questions most commonly asked of us by school practitioners at this point in their exposure to social problem solving.

Aren't These Steps Hard for Children to Learn?

At the heart of life skills teaching, for all youngsters, disadvantaged and advantaged alike, must be the recognition that they stand at the threshold of greater independence and responsibility for their futures [i.e., they stand poised ready to become responsible citizens and contributing members of workplaces, institutions of learning, community, and families]. The decisions they will soon have to make have lifelong consequences for themselves and others; decisions about their education and goals; about smoking, drinking, and drugs; about the use of vehicles; and, tragically, even decisions about the use of weapons. Knowledge [and skills] for the making of judgments can be taught. It is a great mistake to assume that young people will acquire these skills automatically. (Hechinger, 1992, p.128)

The use of an eight-step social problem-solving approach represents a way to consolidate many broad and inclusive skill areas. It also represents our view that students need a social problem-solving *strategy* they can apply in many situations. A reality is that we cannot prepare children for each and every problem and decision and all the ways in which they might occur. The strategy provides *continuity* over time, across experiences with different adults and in different places, and it provides *clarity* amidst the many competing influences on a student's mind. We see the eight-step social problem-solving strategy serving as a beacon in a fog or a lifeline when one is overboard at sea. Indeed, those children who evolve a coping strategy are those most effective in meeting school, home, and peer demands and responsibilities. With the unrelenting numbers of psychological casualties among our students (Bronfenbrenner, 1979; London, 1987), it becomes clear that whatever processes worked in the past to help children become prepared for the roles and responsibilities of adulthood are no longer working adequately. *The eight steps become an explicit, clarifying strategy accessible to all students, not only those skillful enough to extract a useful strategy out of the complex and fast-moving world around them.*

The eight steps are no harder to learn than any other complex set of skills. Recall how you learned to drive a car, do long division, or read a map. When you first learned, you had a step-by-step procedure to follow: "First, you put on your seat belt. Then, you check your rearview mirror. Next, . . ." With time and practice, complex sets of steps and skills go "underground"; they become "routinized" or "automatized" or incorporated into "scripts" or "knowledge networks" (Baron & Brown, 1991; Bransford, Sherwood, Vye, & Rieser, 1986; Perkins, 1986; Sternberg & Wagner, 1986). With experience, the same basic sets of skills are used, except that they become broadened, extended, and further integrated. We never lose sight of the fact that the goal is to build the skills *gradually* so that students possess them when they are ready to emerge into the adult world. There is no expectation that they can be learned, retained, and generalized without a degree of continuing instruction and infusion into academic content and classroom routines. However, as social decision making is taught, children quickly begin to realize the power and usefulness of *thinking*. They come to believe that they can be decision makers and problem solvers. They begin to feel a sense of "I can" that can be built upon even while their skills are being learned. Through a combination of *competence* and *competencies*—the sense of "I can" and the skills to be effective in social problem solving and everyday decision making—we have found we can fortify children against stressors and prepare them for the challenges of their teenage and adult years (Elias, 1989).

How Is This Relevant to At-Risk Students?

We believe that by teaching at-risk children to think carefully and independently through decisions and problems, we will help them see that they have choices, that they have some control over their lives. (Mirman, Swartz, & Barell, 1988, pp. 138–139)

It is becoming recognized that a meaningful part of what puts children "at risk" is a tendency to behave in a way characterized by impulsive decision making that appears to maximize danger and harm to self and others, as well as a certain randomness in thought and action that impairs relationships with peers and adults (Mirman et al., 1988). Yet, instruction in critical thinking and decision making typically is not emphasized for high-risk students (Levine, 1988). The relevance of social problem solving to at-risk students is expressed by Mirman et al. (1988): "The extent to which at-risk students are afforded opportunities to engage in collaborative problem solving may determine whether or not they become less disaffected with the school" (p. 145).

Engaging in problem solving and decision making of the kind described in this book provides at-risk students with a strategy that can correct the flaws or "bugs" in their decision-making process and highlight for them the relevance and benefits of mastering their feelings and pursuing goals in a focused, thoughtful way. Reducing risk status is a matter of increasing both the confidence and competence of students. A social problem-solving approach provides skills and reflects an empowering attitude that students and educators can use to find elements of school that can be meaningful and engaging to students.

Can Social Problem Solving Really Make a Difference in Education and in Students' Lives?

> Decision makers play the roles of philosopher, scientist, designer, and builder. Schooling focused on decision making, the developmental and critical thinking skills that serve it, and the knowledge base that supports it, will allow students to learn these roles, to claim their capacity to think and their heritage as human beings. (Wales et al., 1986, p. 41)

Social problem solving is not a panacea. It is an approach that can be of assistance at various levels. The eight steps have diagnostic value in helping educators uncover areas of strength and weakness. Educators can use the eight steps as part of a strategy to assist them in their own decision-making processes. With students, even on a short-term basis, such as during the course of one academic year with one's class or a special group, there has been evidence of successful use of social decision making and related approaches (Elias, 1983; Kazdin & Associates, 1987; Spivack, Platt, & Shure, 1976). Finally, the best results appear to reflect the same features as for other academic areas: they occur when there is continuity over a period of years, reinforcement and application of skills at times other than during formal lessons, and support from school personnel at a variety of levels (Weissberg & Elias, 1993). We have seen the approach make a difference in a number of school contexts, but always in relationship to the goals and scope defined by the educators involved.

What Elias and Clabby (1992) describe as second generation social problem-solving programs meet the above criteria. These programs, delivered primarily in the form of teacher-led, group-based classroom lessons, focus on a variety of interpersonal skills. Self-control, group participation, and social awareness skills are seen to be prerequisite skills for problem solving. Students learn a decision-making strategy for responding to a variety of everyday difficulties and choices that they face. Finally, social problem-solving programs contain structured activities to ensure generalization of these skills to a variety of academic and social situations. Social problem-solving programs are designed with a focus on the promotion of prosocial interaction and fostering respect for diversity and positive social development for *all* students—both mainstreamed classified students and their nonclassified peers. Classified students can benefit from direct instruction in appropriate social behavior and from *structured and guided* interaction with peers who, on the average, may be more skilled in these areas. Nonclassified students, through ongoing group interaction with classified students, can gain an appreciation of individual differences and learn ways to interact positively with a range of other students.

Is There any Empirical Evidence for Social Problem Solving and Related Intervention Approaches?

Within the school setting, social adjustment is being seen as equally important as academic skill development (Schloss, 1992). Programs that emphasize the development and use of social skills are especially promising for use in inclusive classrooms because they address issues that are relevant to both mildly disordered and nondisordered children. Therefore, social skill instruction, especially procedures incorporating social problem solving, has received extensive empirical study, including longitudinal research (Elias & Clabby, 1992). This section will review several of the most prominent social problem-solving programs.

Shure's (1994) ICPS (Interpersonal Cognitive Problem-Solving, or I Can Problem Solve) has been evaluated over a period of 25 years and more recently in a 5-year longitudinal study. This curriculum is geared toward the promotion of mental health in kindergarten through sixth graders. Designed with "high-risk" children in mind—that is, those who are either impulsive (unable to wait, overly emotional, bossy to peers) or inhibited (overly shy, withdrawn, and passive rather than assertive)—the program includes a pre-problem-solving phase (e.g., identifying feelings and perspective taking) followed by problem-solving training, both of which use games, stories, puppets, and role playing. Results show gains in interpersonal as well as academic behavior, including a reduction in impulsive behavior; however, it is also clear that effects disappear in the absence of "booster" or follow-up sessions.

Like ICPS, Skillstreaming is a method of promoting social skills that emphasizes interpersonal and problem-solving skills. The Skillstreaming Curriculum aims to improve interpersonal communication in prosocial skills such as classroom survival, making friends, dealing with feelings, dealing with stress, alternatives to aggression, and planning (Miller, Midgett, & Wicks, 1992). Skillstreaming relies on modeling, role playing, performance feedback, and transfer of training to promote prosocial skills (Goldstein, Sprafkin, Gershaw, & Klein, 1980). A study by Miller et al. (1992) examined the effects of Skillstreaming on a group of emotionally disturbed students. After using the curriculum for 6 weeks, teachers completed checksheets that examined their perceptions of each student's behavior in the areas of beginning social skills, advanced social skills, dealing with feelings, alternatives to aggression, dealing with stress, and planning skills. Students also completed checklists that rated their personal behavior in the same areas. According to teacher ratings, after receiving the Skillstreaming Curriculum for 6 weeks, middle school students had significantly improved their social skills in all examined areas.

While these and similar programs have shown some success, it has become clear that results tend to be stronger, more generalizable, and enduring as programs are ongoing and long-term (Elias, Weissberg, et al., 1994). Thus, a "second generation" of social problem-solving programs has emerged with a dual emphasis on the integration of the program into the classroom structure and on continuity and reinforcement of skills.

Weissberg's Social Problem Solving (SPS) program (Weissberg, Jackson, & Shriver, 1993) integrates the affective, cognitive, and behavioral aspects of problem solving. Students are taught steps to use when responding to social challenges and problems. These steps are as follows:

1. Stop, calm down and think before you act.
2. Say the problem and how you feel.
3. Set a positive goal.
4. Think of lots of solutions.
5. Think ahead to the consequences.
6. Go ahead and try the best plan.

In a longitudinal study of the program, students who received SPS training were compared to students who did not receive the training. Results indicated that students receiving SPS training showed significant gains in their ability to generate more cooperative solutions to hypothetical problems and endorse assertive and cooperative strategies to resolve interpersonal conflict (Elias & Weissberg, 1990).

Elias and Clabby's (1989) SPS program has been studied since 1979. The program has been delivered to both nonhandicapped and mildly handicapped students in mainstream settings, as well as school-based and residential special education contexts. The scope of the program is multi-year, and those trained in the program learn how to integrate it into all aspects of the school day in an ongoing manner. Major documented effects of the program are that, compared to control groups, children involved in the programs were more sensitive to others' feelings; were seen by their teachers as displaying more positive prosocial behavior; were sought out by their peers more for help with problems; displayed lower than expected levels of antisocial, self-destructive, and socially disordered behavior, even when followed up in high school; and felt that they learned more about their classmates. Also important is that the SPS program has been subjected to external evaluation and has been designated as a program of educational excellence by the Program Effectiveness Panel of the U.S. Department of Education's NDN (Elias & Clabby, 1992).

The Child Development Program (Battistich, Elias, & Branden-Muller, 1992) is another example of an effective SPS approach that seeks to impact on the school environment. The program was designed to create a caring and participatory school community in which children are given opportunities to learn about others' needs and perspectives, to collaborate with one another, and to engage in a variety of prosocial actions, all in balance with their own needs. Group activities include working in small cooperative groups toward common goals in academic and nonacademic tasks. Goals of fairness and consideration are reached through direct training in group interaction skills. Group discussions and meetings are also geared toward increased helping of other students and sensitivity to and understanding of others' feelings, needs, and perspectives.

Results from a longitudinal study of three suburban, middle-class elementary schools (and three control schools) using the Child Development Program indicate that improvement relative to the control group was shown on spontaneous prosocial behavior (helpfulness, support, cooperation), student ratings of the extent to which the classroom was a "caring community", greater ability to take the perspectives of others as well as consider one's own needs, peer acceptance, along with a decrease in loneliness and social anxiety.

Are All Children Ready to Learn the Social Problem-Solving Steps?

> For students to learn to communicate and to function in a social world that is often very different from their own calls for tact and understanding on the part of those who teach life skills. Because words and ideas often have different meanings for teachers and the taught, the first task is to create mutual understanding without impatience or embarrassment. Students must be listened to and treated with respect [and must learn to do the same for others]. (Hechinger, 1992, p. 128)

In the initial years of the Project, the ISA-SPS team followed conventional wisdom and began our program with instruction in the eight decision-making and problem-solving steps. This came to be referred to as the Instructional Phase, and this was followed with a series of lessons and activities designed to foster application of the social problem-solving process to everyday interpersonal and academic situations. The latter series of lessons are referred to as the Application Phase (Elias & Clabby, 1989). As the ISA-SPS team began working with early elementary schoolaged children, special education populations, and children at risk for poor adjustment, two sets of skills were found that appear to be prerequisites for effective social problem solving.

Self-control skills are necessary if students are to effectively monitor interpersonal situations, accurately extract information, and remain involved in the situation long enough to begin to access and use their decision-making abilities. These skills include listening and remembering, following directions, calming oneself when under stress, and starting and maintaining a socially appropriate conversation.

Social awareness and group participation skills reflect the perspective that groups or classes learn and function best as problem-solving teams (Slavin, 1990). Therefore, social problem-solving instruction tends to occur in group situations, using cooperative learning methods (D. Johnson & Johnson, 1990). Key skills include asking for and receiving help, giving and receiving praise and criticism, selecting praiseworthy friends, showing caring, perspective taking, and sharing with the group. Lessons and activities covering these skill areas are part of what is called the Readiness Phase, which typically is an initial target for work involving early elementary and high-risk populations (Elias & Clabby, 1989). The inclusion of the Readiness Phase has led to increased effectiveness of the overall program and extended its scope to be relevant to more diverse groups of students. Indeed, in some districts, children focus mainly on self-control and social awareness skills and do not emphasize the social problem-solving steps (Hett & Clabby, 1993).

A LOOK AHEAD

We share a perspective summarized by Perry London in the *Phi Delta Kappan*:

> For the common good, a sane society needs to educate its citizens in both civic virtue and personal adjustment. . . . The schools must become more important agents of character development, whose responsibility goes beyond such matters as dress, grooming, and manners. Their new role must include training for civility and civic virtue, as well as a measure of damage control for personal maladjustment. (1987, p. 67)

Social problem-solving skills can—and, we feel, must—be built into the way in which schools educate children. There is no doubt about the important role that parents and guardians play and the need to encourage them to meet the responsibilities of that role as diligently as possible (Elias, 1989). However, the urgency of a school-based effort is clear as one considers the nature of school populations, the needs of an increasingly service-oriented and technological culture, and the mission of schools as the primary common, public socializer of children. School practitioners of all disciplines have a critical role to play, by virtue of the nature of their positions, backgrounds, and training, in actualizing this considerable responsibility. The remainder of this book details procedures and activities to help school practitioners bring social problem-solving skills to all students.

CHAPTER 2

♦♦♦

Key Intervention Techniques

♦

The questions we, as thinkers, can pose before, during, and after our engagement with problem solving are designed to affect our control over our own thinking. . . . Why such a strategy would be effective with at-risk students should by now be obvious: by definition, they have little sense of competence within school; they are detached and unmotivated, and see little connection between their "real" lives and what goes on in school. Empowering all students with ways of planning their approach to a problem ("What is my problem? How will I solve it?"), monitoring their progress ("How well am I doing?"), and evaluating their success ("Have I finished? How well have I done?") should, ultimately, affect the conduct of their lives both in and out of school.

—*Mirman et al. (1988, p. 146)*

One of the difficulties in facilitating problem solving and decision making is that we walk a fine line between instruction and counseling. Many teachers are comfortable with the didactic portions of a social skills program but are less familiar with a facilitative approach. The following "Guiding Principles" were developed to encapsulate the most effective way for facilitators to interact with students during problem-solving sessions (see Table 2.1).

GUIDING PRINCIPLES

The Facilitative Approach

The leader of a problem-solving and decision-making group is not there to solve the child's problem or to make the child's decision for them. Lead-

TABLE 2.1. Guiding Principles

1. The facilitative approach
2. Prompting and cuing the skills learned previously
3. Modeling
4. Open-ended questioning
5. The two-question rule
6. The Columbo technique
7. Paraphrasing
8. Patience and persistence
9. Flexibility and creativity

ership of this type of group requires the use of a facilitative approach. This is different from what adults more commonly do. Facilitators are not "experts," imparting their information to the child, nor are they counselors providing potential solutions to the child.

The facilitative approach involves asking questions rather than telling. Also inherent in this approach is a nonauthoritarian manner. It is necessary to step back and allow children to think through the problem, set their own goals, and decide their own course of action. The purpose of social decision making is to help children get what *they* want rather than what the teacher, parent, or peer may want. Skillful guidance through social decision making can help children see that antisocial behaviors do not in fact get them what they really want, which is usually peer acceptance, material enhancement, or getting some adult off their back.

This can naturally make adults uncomfortable because they perceive this as a loss of control or abdication of authority, which it is not. The leader controls and guides children through the process but the leader must be willing not to have a preconceived notion of what the "right" answer is. This will only stifle children's thinking. If children are resistant and the leader is trying to lead them to the "right" answer, they will frustrate the leader. If the children are cooperative, they may give the adult what they want to hear and then not act on it. If the children are compliant, they may carry out an appropriate solution but are not being taught how to become independent problem solvers. (Ways to help teachers and other school professionals feel more comfortable with this approach will be presented in Chapter 8.)

However, it is recognized that due to the less structured less traditional way of leading this type of group, some children will misread this as an opportunity to engage in inappropriate behavior. It is often necessary to have a parallel behavior management program in place to address these problems and keep the discussion and behavior within bounds (see Chapter 3.)

Another concern mentioned by adults is that facilitating problem solving and decision making is value-free. In other words, when the child says that his goal is to rob the convenience store, the leader does not immediately reprimand the child or call the police. Technically, what the leader should do is clarify to the child that robbing the store is something he or she can do to achieve a goal but it is not really a goal in itself. If the goal is to have a lot of money, the leader should help the child think of other things that can be done to achieve this. Then, when "envisioning outcomes for each option," the leader can ask what might happen if the child robs the convenience store. At this point, if the child has not already thought of it, the leader can envision the child going to jail and can point out to the child that when someone is in jail, it is hard to make a lot of money, which was the child's goal. The leader who takes time to help the child think through this kind of scenario rather than reprimanding the child will be much more effective the next time an issue like this comes up.

If the leader takes the role of authority or censor, children will not buy into the process. Adolescents are especially wary of others telling them what to do. Children and adolescents will often bait adults with inappropriate responses waiting patiently for the adult to bite, causing the discussion to get off the topic or end up in an argument. If the adult can establish the general current in terms of the process of problem solving, then the child will be swept along and caught in the net of his own ineffective problem-solving approaches.

Prompting and Cuing the Skills Learned Previously

After skills have been taught, it is necessary to promote generalization. One way to get children to use skills more independently and spontaneously is to remind them. In order to do this, it is helpful to use a prompt or simple way of indicating to the child that now would be a good time to use the skills they learned previously. The readiness skills covered in Chapter 3 have names such as "Keep Calm" or "BEST" that serve as cues to use a set of skills. For example, Keep Calm is a relaxation exercise that can be used when children need to settle down from an overstimulating experience or when they are anxious.

By using a simple prompt, the leader does not have to stop the action and review the whole set of skills involved. In addition, others in the children's environment can be taught the prompt and when to use it without needing full training in how to facilitate social skills; the more pervasive the prompting of skills, the better the generalization will be. In schools, lunch aides can be taught to encourage students to use Keep Calm rather than yelling at them to sit down and shut up. This can be a more positive and effective intervention.

Modeling

Modeling is important because it allows the child to learn by watching the adult use these skills. Seeing the adult utilize the problem-solving skills is much more effective than just telling the child what to do. It is unfortunate that often adults do not let the child in on their thought processes. Letting children in on the adult's thoughts can let children know that it is normal to have negative feelings, be confused, and not have the perfect solution right at your fingertips. It also shows children that you can think your way out of a problem.

The leader needs to find ways of modeling aspects of the program. When introducing a skill, the leader can discuss when he/she used the particular skill. Or when a decision is confronting the leader, he/she can use FIG TESPN to help arrive at a plan. Obviously, this self-disclosure needs to be conducted appropriately, and it should be done without revealing truly personal information.

For example, in a classroom, a teacher may be considering what kind of test to give the students. The teacher may verbalize his/her thought process using FIG TESPN as follows:

"Let's see . . . I'm feeling a little uncertain [feeling] about what kind of test to give you [problem]. I really want to make sure you know the material [goal]. I could give you a take home test [option] but then this would have to be really hard [outcome]. We could do some cooperative learning in teams [option] and that might help you learn to work together better [outcome]. Or, we could just do a regular test [option] but I hate grading those [outcome]. Maybe I'll have you work in groups and the group will receive a grade on the test [solution]. We can have the test next Thursday. It will cover Chapters 3 and 4. I'll give you a set of questions and divide you into groups to answer them [plan]. Gee, maybe some of you will think it's unfair if some students do all the work or if some do a poor job and the whole group gets a low grade as a result [pitfall]. Well, class, what do you think we should do if that happens?"

Open-Ended Questioning

There are four types of questioning: closed-ended questioning ("Did you hit him?"), interrogative questions ("Why did you hit him?"), multiple-choice questioning ("Did you hit him because he was teasing you or because of something else?"), and open-ended questioning ("What happened?"). Closed ended questions require a "yes" or "no" or other one-word response from children, and elicit neither much reflection nor much information. If one asks, "Are you angry?" much less information will be elicited than if the question is phrased in an open-ended manner such as, "What feelings are you having?" On the other hand, most children have difficulty answering "why" questions. This is often because there is an underlying accusation of guilt, and children, like most people, become defensive when they feel blamed. It is also the case that children, in particular, may not be aware of the deep reasons behind their actions; this is especially true of children with behavioral and emotional difficulties.

Nevertheless, there is a strong pull for adults to ask "why" questions in problem situations. In response to, "Why did you hit him?" very few children will say, "Because I have poor emotional control and tend to act impulsively rather than consider alternative actions that may be more effective in solving the problem in the long run," or "I think it stems from repeated exposure to parental discord, which has served to model an aggressive or at times physically preemptive, misguidedly self-protective coping approach on my part. And I watch a lot of violent television without adult supervision, which recent research suggests will exacerbate any violent tendencies I already have." If only children spoke in accurate diagnostic formulations!

Given these limitations in children, adults need to retrain themselves to ask open-ended rather than closed-ended or interrogative questions. A good first step is to practice ways of reframing "why" questions. Some examples are:

"What happened?"
"What did you want to have happen?"
"What were you trying to do?"
"How are you feeling?"
"What was the other person doing?"
"What happened before this?"

Adults sometimes are quick to give multiple-choice questions, especially if children tend to be resistant. Adults usually can make a good guess as to what the possibilities are and present them in a succinct format. However, the goal in social decision making and problem solving is to have children become competent and independent thinkers. For this to happen, we must give them opportunities to think for themselves and not "rescue" them too soon by cutting down the thinking needed on their part. The exceptions to this are with younger children and when there are time constraints. Younger children will have difficulty verbalizing and may need the prompts provided by multiple-choice questions. Also, using only open-ended questions can be time consuming, especially with resistant children. Therefore, although the rule of thumb is to always use open-ended questions, multiple-choice questions can be considered in some situations. Another way of looking at this is that adults lose nothing by starting with open-ended questions, and then moving to the more common types of questions as needed.

In general, by adults' using open-ended questions, a child's thinking about the problem will be maximized. In addition, the more a child has invested in the problem-solving process, the more he or she will feel ownership of the solution. Open-ended questioning, although more time consuming, will eventually help minimize a child's resistance to carrying out positive coping actions.

The Two-Question Rule

This rule is: "Follow up a question with another question." It reminds the leader to stay in the questioning mode. It will also enable the most information to be brought forth, because it "serves notice" on the children that the leader is genuinely interested in hearing details. For example, the question, "How are you feeling?" can be followed up by, "What other feelings are you aware of?" The question, "What are you going to say when you go up to the lunch aide?" can be followed up by, "How exactly are you going to say it?" An example in an academic context would be following a question like, "What are the ways that the body regulates temperature?" with "How do you know that is true?" Indeed, that particular follow-up probe is especially useful, given the array of misinformation and partial information children pick up through television.

Overall, the more that children talk about the problem or the issues under consideration, the better understanding both the adults and children involved will have. Follow-up questioning helps children clarify their own thoughts and feelings.

The Columbo Technique

This strategy was modeled after the Peter Falk character on television, Lieutenant Columbo. This character is perpetually confused and asks lots of questions in an off-hand manner. He scratches his head and has difficulty understanding. He is nonthreatening and therefore people he is talking to do not get defensive. By pointing out inconsistencies in witnesses' stories or having suspects explain the obvious, he obtains the crucial information to solve the case.

This strategy is particularly effective when working with resistant students. For example, if two students were in a fight and one claims that the other just came up and hit him, the adult might ask, "You mean he just came up and hit you? What is getting into people today? Gee, why on earth would he do that? Let's see if we can figure this out. Where were you? What did you say to him before he hit you?" and so forth. Through this line of questioning, you are never directly challenging the student's statements; indeed, you implicitly accept the basis of what the child is saying, which then allows you to ask for more details that might reveal the illogic to the child's story or enough information in a round about way that the student eventually verbalizes what really happened.

The important aspect of the Columbo technique is the nonconfrontational manner. It is important never to say something like, "Come on, no one just comes over to someone else and hits them at random," even when you know they are not telling the whole truth. It is through gentle persistence that the truth will come out. Again, this can be a time-consuming process but the point is to get the student to think about the situation. With resistant students, the more the adult pushes, the more resistant the child becomes. With the Columbo technique, the adult becomes someone a child can talk to because one is giving the child the benefit of the doubt. From a trusting relationship, truth—even if self-incriminating—is likely to emerge. Other truths, such as painful or embarrassing ones, also are more likely to come out when one has modeled an accepting attitude.

Paraphrasing

This strategy should be familiar to anyone who has had training in communication skills. It is important because it helps speakers feel listened to, understood, and validated. By reflecting back to children what they are saying, the listener lets them know that they are being taken seriously, and they are reinforced for speaking.

Another useful aspect of paraphrasing is that the listener can gently rephrase the child's statements into more accurate or appropriate language. Children often have difficulty stating their feelings. For example, when asked, "How do you feel?" a child might respond, "He's an idiot." This can be paraphrased as, "It sounds like you are really angry with him." It is often necessary to translate the child's rough expression of feelings into more refined and precise statements. This will help the children clarify their own thoughts as well as develop a better problem-solving vocabulary.

Patience and Persistence

As has been mentioned previously, teaching problem-solving and decision-making skills takes a long time. It involves teaching a complex set of skills.

Although all children need to learn these skills, some are more facile than others. Just as some children teach themselves to read and others are dyslexic, some children develop these social skills naturally and others have difficulty reading social cues, comprehending social problems, and expressing themselves in a manner that will enable them to have their needs met. These children are what we call "social dyslexics." Just as a reading dyslexic needs more time and effort devoted to reading instruction, a social dyslexic needs more time and effort devoted to social decision-making instruction. If there was an easy way, we would apply it; unfortunately, long and hard work on these skills seems to be the only way, especially if one wants to solidify and generalize behavioral gains.

Persistence is an important component to any skill-building program. The more problem solving is taught, encouraged, and reinforced, the better chance there is that it will be internalized. Teachers, parents, support personnel, and peers should all be involved in a comprehensive manner for maximum effectiveness.

Flexibility and Creativity

Social skills and social decision making cannot be learned from a textbook; they can only be learned by practice. Any program needs to be adapted to both the child's environment and the individual child. Not only do organizational issues need to be taken into consideration when beginning a program, but the characteristics of the group leader and the children need to be identified and addressed.

The components of the program are presented as generic guidelines to be adapted to the specific circumstances of the setting in which they will be taught. Obviously, cultural differences are one important consideration in adapting the program. Other adaptations need to be based on grade level, type of program (regular, special education, or enrichment), and skill levels of the students.

It has been found that the most successful implementers of this program have also been among the most creative. Many innovations have come from implementers. This is because these people have taken the program and made it their own. They have put their own creative stamp on it. This type of adaptation should be encouraged.

AN EXAMPLE OF THE TECHNIQUES IN ACTION

The following excerpt from a classroom discussion allows one to see how a teacher uses the techniques described in this chapter to build the students' skills. Be especially alert for examples of facilitative questioning, prompting and cuing the skills learned previously; modeling, open-ended questioning, the two-question rule, paraphrasing, patience and persistence, and flexibility and creativity.

TEACHER: Class, we seem to have a problem today that I'm feeling a little confused about. We need to review for the test but I also was hoping to do some fun projects. I wonder if FIG TESPN could help us with this. Let's see . . . F . . . feelings. . . . Well, I guess I said that I felt confused about what to do. I also will feel disappointed if we don't get to do the fun things I had planned. . . . I also would feel a little guilty if I didn't help you review for the test. Do any of you have feelings about this problem?

TERRENCE: I want to do the fun stuff.

TEACHER: Okay, but that's a goal. Do you have any *feelings* about this?

TERRENCE: I feel that we should do some review and then do the projects.

TEACHER: That might be a good option and we'll think of things to do in a minute but I'm still kind of wondering how you feel about this.

TERRENCE: I hate reviewing for tests, we already know the stuff and we never get to do anything fun.

TEACHER: Okay, that's great, now we have a feeling. Terrence is feeling angry about having to do a review. Any other feelings?

KRISTIN: I feel happy that we might get to do fun stuff.

TEACHER: Good; "happy" is another feeling.

ESTEVAN: I'm a little nervous about the test.

TEACHER: "Nervous." You are coming up with terrific feeling words. Any more feelings? . . . Laura, is that your hand I see?

LAURA: Excited. I'm excited about doing some fun things in class.

GILLIAN: Me, too! I feel the same way.

TEACHER: I expect that many other students feel excited and are looking forward to it also. Okay, now we want to identify the issue. So what's the problem?

SARA: We want to do the fun stuff but we have to review for the test.

TEACHER: "We want to do fun stuff but we have to review for the test." That's one way to say what the issue is. Any others?

LAUREN: Why can't we just do the fun stuff?

TEACHER: I'm glad you're thinking of things to do, but hold onto that idea for just a couple of minutes until we get to that step. So what's our goal?

ANDY: To do fun stuff.

TEACHER: Okay, that's one goal but we have talked about the other goal of reviewing for the test. Since we are all part of the same class, we need a goal we can all agree on.

ANDY: We can study and then do fun stuff.

TEACHER: That's technically a "thing to do" but maybe you can rephrase that as a goal.

ANDY: To study and also do fun stuff.

TEACHER: Great, now that sounds like a goal to me. Does everybody agree with this goal?. . . Let's see, F—feeling, I—identify the issue, G—goal, T—what's T stand for again?

YASMIN: (*looking at the poster on the wall*) Think of many possible things to do.

TEACHER: Let's list them on the board. One . . .

TERRENCE: Do the fun stuff.

TEACHER: Okay (*writes this on the board*). Another thing . . .

RYAN: Study for twenty minutes and then do fun stuff for twenty minutes.

TEACHER: Great (*writes this on the board*). Something else? Remember, part of our goal is to study but we didn't say how yet.

JEFF: Maybe we could do the review at home and just do the fun stuff here.

TEACHER: (*writes this on the board*) Okay . . . how about some more things?

SAMARA: Do the fun things and those kids who need help could come after school.

TEACHER: Okay, that's great. We have four different things we can do. Next, we want to do what?

MICHELLE: Envision!

TEACHER: Right! So the first suggestion was to do the fun stuff. If we do the fun stuff, what do you envision happening?

MICHELLE: We'll fail the test because we didn't review.

TEACHER: Okay, that might happen. What else might happen? . . . Well, would we meet our goal of "to study and do fun stuff"?

NADINE: No, because we only did fun stuff.

TEACHER: Okay, anything else about this option?

MELISSA: I'd be happy if we did fun stuff.

TEACHER: Okay, that's great. I'm glad you reminded us that it's always important to keep in mind the feelings that we have about the various things we think of doing. Let's see, the next option is to study for twenty minutes and then do fun stuff for twenty minutes.

JOHN: We'd meet our goal.

TEACHER: Yes, we might. Anything else?

MICHAEL: What if we needed more than twenty minutes to study?

TEACHER: Hey, you are way ahead of me. That would be a roadblock to this option, wouldn't it? Well, let's keep that in mind. What else do you envision happening?

MICHAEL: We could have fun.

TEACHER: Okay, we could have some fun. Next option, review at home and do fun stuff here. What do you envision?

MOLLY: Maybe when we get home we won't understand something.

LAKEESHA: I already have too much homework.

CHELSEA: I have dance and music lessons when I get home, so I won't have too much time to review.

PETER: I'd rather review on my own and my father can help me.

TEACHER: Great, okay . . . anything else?

BONNIE: Well, what's the fun stuff you said we were going to do?

TEACHER: I'll show you later if this ends up being part of our plan, but for now, let's try to work with all of FIG TESPN. Okay, any more visions? . . . The last thing we thought of doing was to have fun here and some kids who need help come after school. What might happen?

TOM: I'm not coming after school.

TEACHER: Okay, some kids might not come after school for help. What else?

DALIA: I can't come after school because I have dance but I don't need to come anyway.

TEACHER: Okay, what you said brings up another thing that might happen. Some kids might not be able to come after school; and we would need a way to decide who should come and who should not. Anything else? . . . Now we want to S—".

SAMARA: Solve it!

TEACHER: Good, "solve it," or select our best solution. What do you think?

SAMARA: Twenty minutes for fun and twenty minutes for review.

MIKE: Forget the whole thing.

LIZ: That wasn't one of the things we thought of doing!

MEG: Yeah. Let's follow FIG TESPN!

TEACHER: Reviewing a bit is a good idea! Let's quickly remind ourselves of the things we thought of doing and what we envisioned happening (*reviews this*). Well, which one seems like our best solution?

DIEGO: Studying for twenty minutes and having fun for twenty minutes.

JOHN: If we didn't have to do this stupid FIG TESPN we could've already been done studying.

TEACHER: You know, you are really coming up with great points. Taking time to think and problem solve sometimes can be a pain, can't it? Sometimes it seems easier just to rush out there and do something instead of thinking it through first. Well, if you didn't help me think this through, I would have just said we need to review for the test and it would be too bad if we didn't have time to do the fun activities. But because we were able to think it through, it seems reasonable to me to review for half the time and do our fun activities for half the time. What do you think about using FIG TESPN to help us think through the problem?

HARRIS: I guess it was worth doing.

CLIFTON: I like using FIG—it helps me all the time.

TEACHER: I'm happy to hear this. So, what's our plan?

MYRA: Next period, we'll review and then do fun stuff.

AGNES: Maybe we could review by playing Jeopardy.

TEACHER: Hey, that's something we didn't even think of, having fun while we study. I would like some volunteers to work with me to make up a Jeopardy game while the rest of you go over your notes and the chapter. Next period, we'll review the questions from the chapter and any questions you have. After that, we'll play Jeopardy.

HYUN HEE: Does Jeopardy count as review or fun time?

TEACHER: Let me think . . . we are going to put things from the chapter into the Jeopardy game, so Jeopardy counts as review. But if the 20 minutes of review time ends and we are in the middle of a game, you can have the choice of continuing or doing the other activities I had planned. Can you anticipate any potential roadblocks? . . . And what is the last step in FIG TESPN, what does "N" stand for?

SAMARA: Notice what happened.

TEACHER: Good! At the end of the next period, we'll see how our plan worked because we may want to use it again sometime. All of you really did a great job of problem solving and coming to a decision. You know, I feel much less confused than I did when we started. I think we all should use FIG TESPN more often!

STEPS IN THE DEVELOPMENT OF A SKILL

Teaching skills can be broken down into a process of discrete steps. This process can be used regardless of the skill involved and is not dependent on a specific content. It can be used as a generic structure for social decision-making lessons. The steps are presented in Table 2.2.

This structure for teaching skills can be used across content areas and with a variety of target populations. It can be used in the development of readiness and social decision-making skills in children, it can be used with parent groups and families, and it is a useful professional development tool for the consultant to use with staff members.

Determining the strengths and needs of the group is important because this will enable the group leader or consultant to tailor the program to the specific group being addressed. Although a variety of formal assessment tools can be used, direct observation and interview add a true flavor of the individual characteristics. This data collection should lead to determining a skill focus. It is necessary to know where to start. This focus can be a group building experience, a readiness skill, an aspect of the social decision-making program (FIG TESPN), or reinforcement of one of the skills or subskills. There are many levels of learning for each skill and they can always be dealt with more deeply.

TABLE 2.2. Steps in the Teaching of a Skill

- Determine the strengths and needs of the group (or individual) being addressed.
- Select a skill focus.
- Prepare the group by describing situations in which the skill can be used, explain the skill, and elicit a rationale from the group for the importance of the skill; a rationale must be provided before instruction can begin.
- Ask how the group has handled these situations before, what have they used or tried to help them cope.
- Break the skill down into its component parts.
- Teach a prompt or name for the skill to use when cuing the practice of the skill.
- Ask the group to identify situations in which the skill would be useful to them.
- Teach the component parts through modeling.
- Provide hypothetical situations (via stories, videos, role-play vignettes) for guided practice and rehearsal with feedback.
- Encourage use of the skill inside and outside of the session and integrate with other skills when possible; assign homework.
- Begin subsequent meetings with reviews and testimonials to monitor progress, reinforce skills, and determine next area of focus (i.e., cycle back to beginning of process).

As emphasized, a rationale for the skill must always be presented. People always need to know why they are doing something, what the purpose is, how it fits into and is meaningful for their lives. Social skills cannot be taught in the abstract; they must be taught in the context of people's everyday lives. The more obvious the connection between "real life" and the skill being taught, the better the likelihood that the skill will be learned and used.

Knowing what the individuals have tried before in similar situations is diagnostic and sets the stage for new learning. This helps identify skills already mastered or areas of skill deficit. If the situation has been handled successfully, the skill used can be reinforced and generalized to other situations. If the outcome was unsatisfactory, the need for a new way of approaching the situation is apparent.

Breaking down any complex instruction into component parts is simply good teaching practice. Although they are often taken for granted, social skills are especially complex. For example, "engaging in conversation" sounds simple enough but it can be broken down into the following component parts:

1. Deciding whom to talk to
2. Thinking of something to say or a topic to talk about
3. Approaching the chosen person in a nonthreatening manner and at an appropriate time
4. Staying at a comfortable distance and making appropriate eye contact
5. Active listening
6. Taking turns and timing your comments
7. Keeping the conversation going
8. Asking relevant questions
9. Assessing the other person's interest in what you are saying
10. Modifying your statements relative to the other person's responses
11. Ending the conversation
12. Assessing whether you want to talk to that person again
13. Planning future contact

Even each of these subskills could be broken down further. For example, ending a conversation may involve the following:

a. Being aware of time constraints
b. Bringing closure to the conversation
c. Being sensitive to the other person's perception of how you end the conversation

    d. Terminating eye contact
    e. Movement away from the other person

Too often, skill levels are assumed. A rule of thumb for working with children is to start from where they are and then progress them to where you want them to be in small, success-based steps. Therefore, it is necessary to break down social skills into these discrete steps to teach them in order to avoid further social failure and rejection. This can also help avoid resistance in children. If the child decides to "talk to them" as a solution to a problem but does not know how to do this, he will fail to reach his goal and will then be more resistant to trying something else next time.

As covered previously, prompts are a shorthand way to remind others to use a particular skill. It is often helpful to let the group come up with a name or to use an individual's words. For example, there are many variations of Keep Calm including "Breathing," "Stay Calm," and "Concentration." By naming a skill themselves, the group is personalizing it.

Asking the group to identify situations in which the skill would be useful promotes generalization. Again, things need to be presented in a concrete manner. Students will not necessarily realize that, for example, a self-calming technique like Keep Calm can be used in a baseball game, before a test, when asking a girl on a date, and to help resist provocations by others. Also, having students say when they are going to use it creates a positive social climate for using the skill. No child wants to be "the only one doing it." When children give public statements about when they are going to use a skill, it helps remove inhibition in others.

As discussed previously, modeling is an important way to teach any skill. Children of any age, and especially those with learning disabilities, benefit from tangible examples of seeing a skill put into action. Modeling can be combined with hypothetical situations. When practicing, it is necessary to give children feedback and guide them through a refinement of the skill. One fun way of modeling and using guided practice is to use a role-play game. If the students are working on a skill such as "anger expression" (our way of making the point that one does not learn to "control" anger as much as to express it appropriately), one can arrange to have situations that make the children angry written on slips of paper and put into a hat or bowl. Humorous situations can be included, as well. Students take turns pulling a paper from the hat, reading the situation, and assigning roles to others; then, it is enacted. Those who do not have parts give feedback to the "angry" person and the role play is repeated if necessary. From activities such as this, children will see models of how to handle anger-inducing situations in different, nonviolent ways.

The purpose of social decision making is for students to use the skills outside the group. This must be planned for rather than assumed. Have others (parents, lunch aides) involved in prompting use of the skills. Give specific homework to use a skill. The worksheet in Table 2.3 may be helpful in conjunction with a homework assignment such as "identify someone's feelings."

Once skills have been artificially broken down into component parts, it is necessary to put them back together into the complex array of skills called "living in the real world." When teaching and practicing skills, they can be taught individually as discrete elements but they then have to be used all together. Think of basketball. You can teach the rules of basketball, dribbling, hook shots, jump shots, passing, and other facets of the game, but you will not know how to play until you know how they all are put together and used in the context of an actual game. Therefore, when encouraging use of skills outside the session, make sure to relate them to other skills that might be needed.

Beginning each meeting with a review and testimonial will reinforce all of the above components of skills building and also encourage children to self-evaluate. Repetition of all of the facets of skill building is essential for ultimate success; review procedures also are diagnostic, to determine what additional skills or subskills need to be worked on in future sessions.

TABLE 2.3. Skill Practice Worksheet

Name:_____ Date:_____

Skill practiced:_____

When did you do this?_____

Where were you?_____

Who else was there?_____

What did you do?_____

What did you observe?_____

How did the others react?_____

What else happened?_____

How would you rate yourself on your use of this skill?
    poor   fair   okay   good   excellent

What would you do differently next time?_____

What skill would you like to work on next?_____

TECHNIQUES TO ENHANCE
SOCIAL DECISION MAKING

The above principles rely on human technology for their success. But there are other kinds of technological aids that can be extremely useful to supplement interpersonal efforts in teaching the social decision-making skills. Written vignettes and paper and pencil worksheets are valuable aids. But when videos are substituted for written vignettes, the practice provided is of a more advanced level and may be more generalizable to everyday interaction. For example, to develop better feelings identification, children can be assigned to read a certain book or story and complete the worksheet in Table 2.4; as a more advanced activity, they can be asked to do the same after watching a certain television show. In this worksheet, students would have to select two main characters and list three different feelings for each. They would also have to indicate how they knew the characters were feeling this way.

As will become clearer in subsequent chapters, children also can take one particular character in the television show and help them solve a problem using FIG TESPN. Children can discuss what other alternatives the character could have used to solve the problem and what the potential outcome might have been as a result. If the group is watching the video in the session, the video can be stopped at a problem situation and the group can discuss potential solutions. Children are also motivated to practice social decision making when producing their own videos. They can develop scripts, produce, direct, and act them out. This activity actually serves a dual purpose. Social problem-solving and decision-making skills will be re-

TABLE 2.4. Analyzing Stories and Television Programs

Main character	Feeling	How could you tell?
1. _____	a. _____	_____
	b. _____	_____
	c. _____	_____
2. _____	a. _____	_____
	b. _____	_____
	c. _____	_____

inforced by the content of the video; in addition, the process of working together to create the video will give rise to many opportunities to engage in both group building experiences and problem-solving situations. More detailed examples of video-based instructional technologies will be covered in Chapter 5. Computer software-related technologies will be presented in Chapter 6.

CHAPTER 3

Classroom-Based Applications: Basic/Readiness Skills Development
♦

When implementing a social problem-solving program, it is useful to build readiness first by establishing individual and social controls. In addition, because the format of the program is interactive and not didactic, the leader of the program must have control over the behavior of the students in a manner consistent with the goals of the program. In other words, students must be induced to cooperate not because they "have to" but because these skills are directly relevant to improving their lives. This nonauthoritarian orientation is sometimes difficult to sell and implement. Also, adults are often uncomfortable with this decreased reliance on authority and the threat of aversive consequence. With these group leaders, it is necessary to build a collaborative relationship and often to provide a great deal of modeling to see that it can be done without chaos. The following strategies and activities can be used to foster a productive social environment.

The students themselves may be unfamiliar and uncomfortable with the group process that is involved in teaching social problem solving. The class will be engaging in group discussion and supporting one another in their problem-solving efforts; they will need to have a sense of safety that comes from mutual respect, a feeling of belonging to the group, and a willingness to share their experiences. In addition, the students will require self-control in the classroom and in other situations where social decision making skills will be used. They will also have to be able to communicate effectively with others in an assertive rather than a passive or aggressive manner. Obviously, these are life skills as well as prerequisites for group participation.

BEHAVIOR MANAGEMENT SYSTEM

Whenever students are engaged in lessons that are less didactic and formal than is typical and students are encouraged to express their ideas openly, there is an increased opportunity for students to engage in inappropriate behavior. The leader must walk a fine line, providing structure and limits for students while at the same time encouraging open expression and independent thinking. Successful social decision making requires students to learn to think for themselves in order to make successful life decisions.

In order to walk that line between limits and freedom, strong consideration should be given to establishing a behavior management system for the classroom. The purpose of this system is to give students feedback on their behavior in terms of what is appropriate and inappropriate and to provide them with consequences that will motivate them to engage in appropriate behavior. The consultant should assess the potential for inappropriate behavior in the students, preferably through record review, leader interview, and direct observation. Although most teachers already have ways of coping with behavior problems, the consultant should have the group leader articulate their behavior management system in order to ensure its effectiveness and consistency with the goals of social problem solving. The consultant should discuss what strategies the leader currently uses with disruptive students. It is possible that no additional strategies are necessary but this will allow the consultant to become familiar with the leader's orientation to this topic. If additional strategies are necessary, group leaders will be more accepting if strategies are presented in a form consistent with the current structure.

The behavior management system should be administered in a matter-of-fact manner and be part of the general classroom routine. Expression of anger by the group leader will be antithetical to the purpose of social decision making and will undermine the effective use of these techniques. The leader should explain the behavior management program to the students prior to implementing it; the leader should emphasize that the purpose of this behavior management program is not to punish. The purpose is to help students respect one another and themselves. It is always important that the rationale for the particular activity be included. Students often assume that any consequence is a punishment for being "bad" rather than a tool to help them learn behaviors that will benefit them in the long run.

The following techniques are derived from work in behavior modification and social learning theory (cf. Braswell & Bloomquist, 1991; Cartledge & Milburn, 1984; Gordon & Asher, 1994; Gresham & Elliott, 1993; Kendall, 1988; Patterson, 1975; and Valentine, 1987, for additional information).

One simple technique that teachers have found to be effective is one minute of detention for each instance of calling out or other inappropriate behavior. Students names are put on the board or on a chart and each time they behave inappropriately, a slash mark is put next to their name. If they protest, another slash mark is put there. It is important for the leader to continue with whatever else was happening in the classroom while slash marks are put up. This is so that the inappropriate behavior will not receive a great deal of leader attention and will not disrupt the general flow of class.

Those behaviors that will warrant a minute of after-school waiting time, or detention, should be delineated clearly to the students. When putting slash marks on the board, no explanation should be given at that time. Discussion should occur either when the program is being set up, or after school before the detention time starts. In schools where detention is not a viable alternative, some other form of punishment should be used that is at least mildly aversive to students and is consistent with school policy.

The second technique found to be useful is similar to the first but in a different form. It can be called "Three Strikes and You're Out." For each instance of inappropriate behavior, the student is given a "strike." When the student has gotten three strikes, he or she is "out." An out earns a "time-out" in the back of the classroom or some other mild punishment. After this the student may continue to collect strikes and outs until he or she has received three outs in the period. At that time, a more severe punishment should be administered such as being sent to the principal, detention after school, a note home to the parents, and so forth. Again, it is important to define those behaviors that will receive strikes, to administer strikes and outs in a calm manner without allowing it to disrupt the class, and to use the technique in a systematic and consistent manner.

Behavior management systems that focus on the group rather than individuals also can be helpful. For example, the leader can establish a baseline rate for inappropriate behavior, such as 10 instances of calling out, rude noises, and put-downs for each period. If the group has less than 10 instances, they earn a choice of activity such as computer time, learning game, and so forth. More than 10 earns them a loss of a privilege. An alternative could be to give 10 minutes towards a special activity each day, which could be redeemed on Friday. Each time any student behaved inappropriately, 1 minute would be taken off. Whatever time was left each day could then be redeemed on Friday when the class could have a special activity or educational game. The leader can be creative in the use of rewards and punishments. Keep in mind that rewards should be pleasurable to students and punishments aversive (e.g., some students dislike educational games and others thrive on the attention they receive in after-school detention).

For older children, techniques involving individualized contracts may be most effective. A contract is an agreement between two or more people that delineates the responsibilities of each party. Simply stated, a contract means, "If you do this, then I'll do that." The leader may wish to introduce the concept of contracts to the class as a whole and generate discussion around the importance of contracts for society. The leader can develop a contract for the class as a whole or for an individual student wherein the class's or student's responsibilities are stated explicitly (assignments completed within the specified time period, homework handed in daily, treating each other and the leader with respect, talking at appropriate times in the classroom, refraining from aggressive behavior, etc.). A system for monitoring the responsibilities will be necessary and should not be so complex that the monitoring is inaccurate or inconsistent. Students can be made responsible for their own monitoring if there is some way of checking the reliability. Of the utmost importance is that the behaviors listed in the contract be precise and clear to all parties concerned.

The next phase of contract development requires negotiation and determination of the leader's or others' responsibilities. Although the students probably "should" be doing the things outlined in the contract, at the present time they may not be motivated to engage in them. Problem students often lack internal motivation to learn because of their frequent experiences with failure. Also, they may not be motivated to please others because of their conflicted social relationships. In these cases, it will be necessary to work with the students to identify what is motivating to them. The "Premack Principle" may be useful here; this principle states that activities that are voluntarily engaged in frequently can be used to reinforce behaviors that are infrequently engaged in. For example, a student who spends his/her free time in shop class can be allowed extra shop class if he/she has completed assignments in other classes.

It is important that the group leader and student negotiate the terms of the contract. A contract that is imposed on the student will not be successful. It is necessary for the student to feel that he/she bas been a part of its development in order for him/her to buy into it. Usually when students feel that they are being listened to by the leader and that their needs are being taken into consideration, they will generate contracts with appropriate terms. Some students will make demands on themselves that go beyond those of the leader. In this case, make sure that the terms of the contract are obtainable. Inclusion of the student in contract development is consistent with the philosophy and practice of social problem solving.

Once the behaviors required of the student, the contingent leader behaviors, and the method of monitoring are delineated, it is necessary to draw up a formal, written contract that is signed by all concerned parties. This part of the process makes it more concrete, lets the student know that you will comply with its terms, and emphasizes its importance. Time frames can also be included in the contract so that review and renegotiation occurs on a regular basis.

GROUP COHESION

The next readiness skill area that requires consideration is the cohesiveness of the group. Feelings of trust and tolerance among students allow them to begin to share some of their experiences and benefit from the experiences of others. The group behavior management program described above may be helpful, as students are given motivation to learn to help one another behave appropriately.

The Sharing Circle

We have found that a vehicle we have called a "Sharing Circle" is an important facet in building a sense of group trust, belonging, and cohesiveness. The Sharing Circle (which need not be a circle, but requires only that the children can face each other as they are speaking) begins as an opportunity for students to say their names and respond to questions that, at first, are innocuous. Some examples of such questions are: "What is the luckiest thing that ever happened to you?"; "What is your favorite restaurant, and what is your favorite thing to order there?"; "What hobbies do you have?" Gradually, the Sharing Circle questions become more personal as the group gets to know and trust one another and it is clear that the classroom rules created are working to "protect" students. Some examples of Sharing Circle topics include telling about your favorite part of your house; something helpful you did for a member of your family; a time during the past week when you worked as part of a team; an example of when you laughed a lot; a time when you wanted to yell at someone or even hit someone, but you stopped yourself. The Sharing Circle might also include questions such as the following: If you could trade lives with a brother, sister, or classmate, would you?; If so, who would you pick, and why?; If you could be invisible for a day, what would you do?; and If you were given $1,000 to use to help other people, how would you spend it?

  Clearly, much thought goes into the pacing and sequencing of these questions. After the Sharing Circle, social problem-solving skills or academic lessons can be introduced. The Sharing Circle is an affirming activity that is an excellent way to start a school day, as a bridge from home concerns; a way to start the afternoon, to help get students focused and oriented for what is to come; and a good way to end the day or week, as a mode of transition and an opportunity to review what went on and what is upcoming.

The Classroom Constitution

Another aspect of group cohesion is a sense of structure, and an effective strategy for developing this is the establishment of a "Classroom Constitution." This teaches students the importance of rules and gives them an experience of group decision making. It is similar to the contract developed with the individual student but can be considered a contract among the group.

Through the Classroom Constitution, students can engage in a democratic and interactive rule-setting process, discuss and develop social norms for classroom behavior, and establish a reference for reminding students of behavioral expectations and prompting appropriate social behavior.

The group leader should first discuss the United States Constitution in a general manner. A review of the vocabulary and concepts related to the Constitution may also be helpful such as: *constitution, article, amendment, law, contract, rights, and responsibilities.*

Next, the group leader can discuss with the students why a constitution is important, that is, what would happen if there was no constitution or law. The ways a constitution would be helpful to the class should also be discussed. Some desirable responses are that a constitution would help maintain order, facilitate respect for one another, establish rules that both student and leader would have to abide by, and enable students to know what is expected of them.

The group leader and students can generate a list of "articles" for appropriate classroom behavior. This list should be wide open and can encompass whatever the students and leader believe to be important. Include both "do's" and "don'ts." All proposed articles should be written down in a brainstorming process and then reviewed and edited.

The leader should review the final Classroom Constitution with the students and take a vote to adopt the constitution. It should be indicated that this will now be the "law" of the classroom. Obviously, the constitution can be amended if the need arises, in other words, if further clarification or additional rules are necessary. The leader can also inform students that he/she will act as Supreme Court, which holds the responsibility for interpreting the constitution (this will reassure the leader that there is no separation of power here). If students reject the constitution, the leader can explain to them that the alternative to a democracy is a dictatorship and that the leader will gladly serve as dictator if they do not wish to exercise their democratic rights.

The students can engage in several activities that expand upon the Constitution:

1. Have students make copies of the constitution. They can use fancy lettering or the computer if available. They can include an eagle or some other symbol to embellish a document.
2. Make a classroom poster of the constitution. This can be a group project.

When developing the constitution, attempt to state rules in a positive manner. For example, instead of "Don't interrupt," the rule may be phrased, "Students have the right to speak and be listened to by others." The initial generation of the rules should be without censorship or criticism. When editing them into a final version, try to get a consensus.

State rules as specifically and behaviorally as possible. For example, "Be nice to others" can be defined as not talking out of turn, asking permission to borrow something, and so forth. Specifics can be generated by asking "What would 'nice' look like?" or "If you were being 'nice,' what would or wouldn't you be doing?"

Subsequent to this lesson, when rules are violated, remind students of the constitution (sometimes just by pointing to it) and remind them that they generated the rules and agreed to abide by them. This can be done in a matter-of-fact manner, such as, "Article 5 of our constitution states that students will refer to other students by their proper names or commonly accepted nicknames (rather than 'stupid' or 'jerk')." If the class exists intact over a period of several years, a constitutional convention can be called at the beginning of the year to review and revise the constitution as necessary. The consultant may need to prompt the leader to continue to refer to the constitution throughout the year, revising it as necessary; often it is noted that leaders set up excellent behavioral guidelines but lack adequate monitoring and follow through.

Peer Activities

Other group building exercises can involve the class as a whole on a project, requiring each person or subgroups of children to complete a part. Students can engage in peer teaching or peer tutoring activities where they help one another learn and grades are assigned based on how much each team has learned pre- to posttest. Several books are listed in the reference section that give details of how to implement these techniques. For example, groups of students can be assigned to be different countries. Each student in the group is given a certain area of expertise to develop: history, economics, political system, art and culture, and so forth. The students could either research their area on their own or be given materials by the leader. Students would then be required to teach the others in their group about their area and the group as a whole would make a presentation to the class. Students could be tested on three levels: their individual area, knowledge of the country, and knowledge of all the countries. This type of learning also has applications to drug and sex education curricula.

Another method of peer teaching is to divide the class into teams that need to master a certain amount of material. The teams can then compete in television game-show formats such as Jeopardy with each member of the team taking a turn to answer. It is necessary for the more advanced students to help the less advanced ones in order to win. This has been found to help all levels of students learn at a faster rate. Groups of students can be assigned problems to solve, social experiments to conduct, class presentations, and so forth that require cooperation and coordination among students. Grading can be based on the groups' overall performance as well as the degree of cooperation and equal division of responsibilities.

SELF-CONTROL SKILLS

Perhaps the most difficult but most important instructional task is that of teaching self-control and proper communication skills. Children may have effective social decision-making and problem-solving skills and, in certain circumstances, be able to put them to make positive use; however, without adequate self-control and assertiveness, they may act impulsively or succumb to peer pressure. For example, even though students are taught the dangers of drugs and can verbalize worthwhile social values, they may not translate these into thoughtful behaviors when confronted with pressures from within or without.

Keep Calm

The Keep Calm activity, derived from Elias and Clabby (1989), is designed to help students stop and think prior to acting. It is a means of reducing impulsivity and giving students a chance to separate their emotional reaction from their cognitive and behavioral reaction. This can then enable them to act based on thoughtfulness, in addition to affective information.

The following are the objectives of Keep Calm:

1. To point out problematic situations where self-control can be used to calm the student down before reacting.
2. To teach students, through a deep breathing and stress-distracting exercise, how to get calm and keep their self-control in a problematic situation.
3. To practice a deep breathing and stress-distracting exercise.

The Keep Calm exercise can be taught to students at any time and in both formal and informal settings. However, optimally, it should be taught, practiced, and reinforced before the need has clearly arisen. If students have practiced this exercise in less stressful situations, they are more likely to use the skill in vivo. To begin this exercise, it should be explained to students that, at one time or another, everyone finds themselves in a conflict or problem situation that needs to be solved. These can be problems in school, or problems with other students, a teacher, parents, or friends, and so forth. Sometimes we might jump right into trying to deal with the problem before we are ready. The Keep Calm exercise is to learn how to stay calm and keep self-control in a conflict situation so that we are ready to deal effectively with the problem.

The leader should begin by asking the children what it means to use *self-control*. Ask them to tell of different *times* and *situations* in which they have to use self-control. Then, ask for ways they *show* self-control, or *things they do* to keep self-control. The group leader should put these examples on the board.

Children need to understand that our bodies send us signals that we are about to lose our self-control. These signals are signs of feeling upset and are called Feelings Fingerprints. Some people get headaches, nervous stomach, stiff neck, or sweaty palms. Leaders can model for the class situations where they felt upset and what their Feelings Fingerprints were. Students can generate examples of situations that they felt upset and what their Feelings Fingerprints were. Those situations are labeled as "Trigger Situations." The leader should list the Feelings Fingerprints on the board and emphasize that Feelings Fingerprints are helpful because they warn us that we are in a tough situation and need to use our self-control to keep calm.

The students can be told that when someone bothers them, when they are in a tough situation, when they are in some other Trigger Situation, or when they notice their Feelings Fingerprints, it is important to Keep Calm before trying to solve the problem.

A Keep Calm handout can be created and distributed to the class (see Table 3.1); as an additional cue, posters can be put up in classrooms or group rooms.

TABLE 3.1. Keep Calm

Keep Calm is something that will help you get ready to solve problems and handle your Trigger Situations. There are four simple steps to remember.

1. Tell yourself, "Stop and take a look around."
2. Tell yourself, "Keep calm."
3. Take a deep breath through your nose while you count to 5, hold it while you count to 2, then breathe out through your mouth while you count to 5.
4. Repeat these steps until you feel calm.

Keep Calm works to produce self-control in three stages:

1. Repetition of the Keep Calm steps out loud with the leader prompting use of each step individually.
2. Repetition of the Keep Calm steps to oneself in a whisper and using the entire procedure when prompted.
3. Silent and spontaneous repetition of Keep Calm by the student.

A way of practicing Keep Calm is to have the class read the Keep Calm steps out loud. Then, have someone lead the group in some physical activity that can be performed at one's seat (jumping jacks, running in place, etc.). After one or two minutes of activity, say to students, "All right, let's use Keep Calm. Say 'stop and take a look around' . . . say 'keep calm' . . . take a deep breath through your nose while counting to 5, hold it to a count of 2, breathe . . . out through your mouth to a count of 5. How many of you are starting to feel calm?" (As necessary, repeat Keep Calm.)

For the second stage, use a similar physical activity, except start the children by saying, "When I say 'Now,' use Keep Calm to calm yourselves down. Say the Keep Calm in a whisper. Look at the poster if you forget the steps."

At the third stage, when the class returns from lunch, recess, gym, or some other activity that is unsettling, ask the class to use Keep Calm silently. Develop signals or cues for the children to use to tell you when they are calm.

It is important for adults to continue to prompt the use of Keep Calm when a child is upset or beginning to lose control; it can also be used prior to tests, school plays, or any other anxiety-provoking or trigger situation. (For older students, situations such as school dances, job interviews, and peer pressure to try dangerous or antisocial actions are times to use Keep Calm.) The greater the number of staff members staff involved in prompting students to use Keep Calm and other social problem-solving strategies, the more quickly students will master them. Therefore, as an adjunct to the main program, a range of school staff (e.g., lunch aides, gym teachers, vice-principals, bus drivers) can be coached in these strategies.

The following scripts can be used by all school personnel:

"Use your Keep Calm steps."
"Stop and think about what's happening."
"Can you feel your Feelings Fingerprints?"
"Let's use Keep Calm and calm ourselves down."
"Let's take a look at what's going on. Tell me what happened, how you are feeling, . . ."
"Take another deep breath and relax and then we can talk about it."

In the classroom program, Keep Calm can be reinforced through several activities. Have students keep a list of situations that are coming up or that they can anticipate in which using Keep Calm will be helpful to them. Also have them keep track of when Keep Calm should have been used. Present students with situations and rehearse and practice preparing for difficult situations or for getting upset and using Keep Calm.

Some students, especially older ones, may balk at using Keep Calm. For these students, it can be helpful to introduce Keep Calm as an exercise developed by sports psychologists and managers of musicians of all kinds to enhance athletic and musical performance. Discuss with them anxiety-provoking situations (asking someone for a date, going for a job interview) and how anxiety interferes in performance. Ask them to watch athletes (baseball batters hitting in a clutch spot, basketball players taking a foul shot, and Olympic divers give especially good demonstrations) prior to performing a feat that requires concentration and skill in the face of stress. Have the students notice that the athletes take a breath or engage in a self-calming activity. This is exactly what Keep Calm is. (An example with musicians can be used instead or in addition.) Then, try to have them connect these points to their own social and academic "performances."

Self-Verbalization

Another technique that fosters self-control and the inhibition of impulsivity is the use of self-verbalization. For example, when having difficulty with something, people tend to talk themselves through it. The leader can model this technique for students numerous times during the day whenever it is necessary to make a decision. It is also beneficial to let students in on adult thought processes, from which they can learn a great deal. Also encourage students to verbalize what they are thinking. Enlist students in sharing times they or their friends "talked themselves through" some problem or decision. It is often necessary to use the facilitative questioning method described in Chapter 2 to encourage students to do this. The process of this kind of dialog, however, results in a strong individual and classroom sense of "I can."

BEST Behavior

In addition to external controls (behavior management, group cohesion) and internal controls (Keep Calm, self-verbalization), it is also necessary for students to assert themselves and exercise appropriate controls on their environment through effective communication. The group leader should be aware of the following:

1. Students need to distinguish between passive, aggressive, and confident styles of behavior.
2. Students need to distinguish passive, aggressive, and confident styles in the following four components of "BEST" behavior:

   B—**B**ody posture
   E—**E**ye contact
   S—**S**aying appropriate things
   T—**T**one of voice

BEST refers to a way of communicating with others that enables someone to be sure of themselves and increase the chance of being understood and respected by others. (BEST was adapted from Elias and Clabby's [1989] equivalent VENT acronym and lesson activity, with the assistance of Linda Bruene-Butler.)

Have the group leader explain that there are three different ways one can communicate with another person. These can be called the Blaster (aggressive), the Shrinker (overly passive), or the Me (effective). The Blaster is aggressive, pushy, and bossy towards others. Blasters act like they do not care about other people's feelings and try to get what they want by bullying others. The leader can help students anticipate what might happen if Blasters try to get what they want in an aggressive way. Although they may sometimes get what they want, others will not like them and this may interfere with their ability to get what they want in the long run.

The Shrinker is meek and passive. Shrinkers seem to care more about what others want than what they themselves want. Shrinkers do not stand up for themselves or really try directly to get what they want. Shrinkers seem to let others walk all over them. Have the leader help the

students understand that although Shrinkers avoid conflict, they also usually do not get what they want.

Obviously, the Me is the best of both the Blaster and the Shrinker.
Me's know what they want and are not afraid to ask for it. However, they
take into consideration other people's feelings and their rights, as well.
Me's say what they feel but in such a way that others can listen to them.
Me's know they can't have what they want all the time, but that the best
way to get what they want most of the time is to work with others.

BEST is a way of helping students act more like a Me rather than a
Blaster or a Shrinker. It stands for:

B—**B**ody posture: standing up straight, being confident in yourself
but not arrogant.

E—**E**ye contact: looking the person directly in the eye, communicating with them openly.

S—**S**aying appropriate things: using appropriate language and saying
what you really feel.

T—**T**one of voice: using a calm voice, not whispering or shouting.

Cultural variations in BEST behaviors are extremely important to
take into consideration. Students should discuss differences around eye
contact (posture, etc.) and discriminate where and with whom different
types of eye contact (posture, etc.) are most and least useful. An interesting
class research project is to have them do multicultural Be Your BESTs,
studying and presenting to one another how people of different cultures
might have different ideas about aspects of BEST skills.

Especially valuable is to have the class think of situations where they
could use BEST. Throughout the social problem-solving process, it is helpful to have group leaders selectively self-disclose situations when they have
used some of these skills. Generate several scenarios and have students act
out Blaster, Shrinker, and Me behaviors. While some students are role
playing, assign other students to watch them and give feedback on the four
components of BEST. Practice can continue until improvement is noticed,
and then others can have a turn.

Older students find the BEST skills relevant but are less likely to relate to the Blaster, the Shrinker, and the Me. However, they can generate
examples of "too much" and "too little" BEST behavior and then create
their own labels. It is often useful to introduce BEST in the context of a
common class or group problem, such as talking to friends, dating, entering a group, job and other interviews, or starting new situations like camp
or after-school clubs or sports. Older students especially enjoy the multicultural Be Your BEST activity. Table 3.2 contains some additional BEST
practice activities.

TABLE 3.2. Additional "Be Your BEST" Activities

Discuss, role play, or write about the following situations and possible responses.

1. You spot your best friend coming out of a movie theater with another friend. Earlier in the day, she told you she had to visit her aunt. You are feeling hurt. How should you handle this situation?

   a. I would not say anything to her because she might get angry at me.

   b. I would mention it to her in order to hear what she had to say.

   c. I would call her later and really let her have it for leaving me out. I may ignore her for a few days also and tell all my friends to ignore her, too.

2. A classmate borrowed $2.00 from you and hasn't paid you back. It has been 3 weeks. How should you handle this situation?

   a. I would give him a piece of my mind and say that if he does not pay, he'll be sorry.

   b. I would not bother him and hope that he pays one of these days.

   c. I would remind him again and ask him when he will have the money.

For the following situations, indicate whether the person is acting like a Blaster, Shrinker, or Me. If the person is acting like a Blaster or Shrinker, role play a Me. If the person is a Me, see if the students can think of other ways of acting like a Me for the situation.

1. John/Jean has been bothered by a boy/girl in his/her class. For some reason, he/she keeps picking on him/her. John/Jean sees the other boy/girl coming. He/she quickly starts walking in the other direction to avoid him/her. How is John/Jean acting? What else could he/she do?

2. Marie's/Martin's mother has been very angry at her/him lately. Today Marie/Martin forgot to take out the garbage and her/his mother grounded her/him for 2 days. Marie/Martin had really been looking forward to a going to a party with friends that night. She/he went to her/his mother, apologized, and offered to help with some cleaning. She/he also promised to leave a note to her/himself on her/his desk to remind her/him about taking the garbage out next time. How is Marie/Martin acting? What else could she/he do?

CHAPTER 4

FIG TESPN:
A Skill-Based Classroom
and Group Intervention
♦

FIG TESPN is an acronym for the sequence of steps that guides students through the process of social decision making and problem solving (see Table 4.1). It provides a centralizing concept for students to understand the steps as a whole process to engage in when confronted with a problem or decision. The unique "name," FIG TESPN, is also a mnemonic that reinforces memory. In addition, it is a convenient prompt for teachers to use; for example, they can ask a student, "How can FIG TESPN help you with this problem?"

This model was developed to be implemented in a flexible manner across a broad variety of settings. Rather than a set of eight discrete steps to problem solving, FIG TESPN is taught as a whole process. It is through the repetition of the whole that the skills embedded within it are learned without losing the overall purpose of solving the student's problem. Each time the process is repeated, a subskill (such as identification of feelings, goal setting, role playing assertive behaviors, etc.) can be highlighted and reviewed.

FIG TESPN can be thought of as "Jiminy Cricket," the character from *Pinocchio* who sits on Pinocchio's shoulder, or like a coach who helps you develop skills but ultimately has to stay on the sidelines. Although FIG TESPN, initially with the leader's assistance, guides the student through the problem-solving process, the student is responsible for generating the ideas that will be used in the process. It is important for the facilitators to keep in mind that the overall goal is to develop students' independent and responsible problem solving. The following are some of the important features of each problem-solving step.

TABLE 4.1. FIG TESPN, Social Problem Solver

1. **FEELINGS** cue me to problem solve.
2. **I** have a problem.
3. **GOALS** give me a guide.
4. **THINK** of things to do.
5. **ENVISION** outcomes.
6. **SELECT** my best solution.
7. **PLAN** the procedure, anticipate pitfalls, practice, and pursue it.
8. **NOTICE** what happened and now what?

Feelings cue me to problem solve. Feelings are the first step in problem solving because they provide a cue that something needs to be done. Often when students have negative feelings, they get stuck in those feelings and become immobilized or act out inappropriately. FIG TESPN teaches them to use these feelings, not as an end result of some unpleasant event, but as a beginning to help them get what they want. A useful analogy is physical pain. If someone got a cut and it did not hurt, they might not notice and could bleed to death or get an infection. The pain from the cut lets them know that there is a problem and that they need to do something to take care of it. If they do not take care of this problem, then things will probably get worse. Bad feelings work the same way. Being upset lets you know that there is a problem that needs to be solved; if you do not solve it, it will most likely get worse. By using feelings as the cue to problem solving, the bad feelings get reframed and students become empowered into action.

It is important to be aware of feelings and identify them. For example, students often do not differentiate between disappointment and anger. By learning to label these feelings appropriately, students are led to different courses of action. You do not do the same things when you are disappointed as you do when you are angry. Learning to label these feelings accurately is called "developing a feelings vocabulary."

The facilitator can have students generate a feelings vocabulary to help expand their awareness. Students can be taught to identify feelings in others (review of the BEST behaviors can be useful here) through facial expression, body posture, voice, and so forth. A fun exercise is to play feelings charades where a student picks a feeling from a hat, acts it out, and the others guess what it was.

I have a problem. This does not mean that the problem was the student's fault, but it does mean that it is the student's responsibility to solve it. Students often externalize blame and thereby externalize responsibility for solving the problem. This then leaves the student powerless to impact on the problem. The purpose of this step is not to ascribe blame but to have the student put the problem into words, which is the first step in solving it. Problems cannot be solved at the feeling level; this step begins to introduce a cognitive process that can lead to solutions.

It is important to identify the problem and sort it out from the various other problems or feelings that may be occurring. Having students verbalize a problem is another technique for fostering impulse control through self-verbalization. At this point, if students come up with problems that seem to be irrelevant to a situation, do not censor them or direct them to the "correct" problem. Allow them to continue through the subsequent steps. At some point, they may see that their solution does not address the problem as stated. At that point, go back and reformulate the problem.

For example, two students had a fight. The teacher asks what the problem is. One student says that the problem is that John is a jerk. The student then attempts to develop goals and options to deal with this. He may see that regardless of what his goal or solution is, he is not addressing the fact that John is a jerk. At that time, you may help the student reformulate the problem, such as "John keeps teasing me."

Goals give me a guide. This step involves turning the problem upside down into a positive statement of desired outcome. The purpose of FIG TESPN is for students to get what they want. However, it will be necessary for students to set appropriate and obtainable goals.

At this step, students should define what a goal is (e.g., a specific thing you want to accomplish or have happen). The facilitator can explain that goals give us direction so that we can work for something. Clarifying goals enables us to develop plans to reach them. It is important for students to develop reasonable and reachable goals. It may also be necessary to identify subgoals; a student who wants to get an "A" in science must first get an "A" on the next test. Having students define general goals for themselves and discussing them can be a worthwhile activity in itself.

Think of things to do. Students generally do not recognize that there is more than one way to meet a goal. Often, even if they think before they act, they do not necessarily think of multiple things they can do. But the more potential solutions they can generate, the better their chance of getting what they want.

It is necessary to teach students how to brainstorm options. This involves writing down everything they can think of relevant to the problem. When brainstorming, it is important not to be critical in the initial stages because outrageous options may stimulate thought about more realistic ones. After brainstorming, then go through the options and refine or combine them. Refrain from rejecting options based on their potential outcomes at this point. Wait for the next step to help students understand that the option may have unpleasant outcomes for them.

Envision outcomes. After generating a list of things to do, it is necessary to go back over them and envision what would happen if they tried one of them. The word "envision" was chosen carefully to evoke imaging, or seeing in a concrete way what would happen. It is helpful if students picture the outcomes, not just think about them.

The facilitator should discuss with students the importance of anticipating the consequences of actions. Students need to understand that for every action there is a consequence. Have students generate examples of actions and consequences. Encourage students envision of several consequences for each action or option; the use of flow charts or webs can make this more graphic. You may also wish to develop a rating system to evaluate potential outcomes for each option, from positive to negative. Some students have difficulty with this and it may be necessary for the facilitator to suggest potential outcomes that were unforeseen by the students.

Select my best solution. When selecting the best solution, refer back to the original problem and goal. Often, students have become distracted by this point and have lost sight of their original goal. Remind them of what they said they wanted. Make sure that the solution addresses this. It may be necessary to rethink one or several of the previous steps. When formulating a solution, several options can be combined. For example, where the goal is to pass a test, the solution may be to develop a study schedule, ask a friend to study with you, and outline all of the chapters.

Plan the procedure, anticipate pitfalls, practice, and pursue it. There are obviously a lot of important skills packed into this step. If students could just do this step, they would be good problem solvers. That actions can be thought out and planned beforehand is often a new but not necessarily welcomed concept to students. However, it should be emphasized to students that planning gives them a better chance of getting what they want.

Planning is often a difficult step for students and they are not accustomed to thinking in a deliberate manner before acting. The use of relevant analogies to reinforce the importance of this can be helpful: the planning that goes into a space shuttle launch, the planning necessary for a family vacation, planning how and when to ask someone for a date. Plans can be broken down into four components: who, what, when, and where. Make sure plans involve each of these components.

Anticipating pitfalls, roadblocks, or obstacles, to the plan is extremely important. The leader should ask, "What could happen that would prevent you from implementing your plan?" By preparing students ahead of time for these pitfalls, you will be inoculating them to some degree against frustration and feelings of futility.

Practice means role playing. It is necessary to make the practice session as concrete and real to life as possible for students in order to help them generalize these skills to the outside world. Students may be able to tell you what they are going to do but lack the skills to do it. Also, having them act it out enables the leader to assess deficits in behavioral skills such as assertive communication, negotiation, or anger control that may need to be addressed prior to plan implementation.

Pursue it means that students have to go out and try it. They need to make a public commitment to do it. Students need to be specific about when they are going to do it.

Notice what happened and now what? It is important for the leader to follow up with the student as to what happened and to have the student engage in self-evaluation. Did the plan work? How does he feel now? Were there unanticipated obstacles? Was the goal realistic and obtainable?

At this step it is important for students to understand that despite their best efforts, their plans might not meet with success. It is necessary to self-evaluate and, if necessary, to rethink the problem or decision. It may be necessary to engage in another FIG TESPN using the result of the initial FIG TESPN as the problem to be solved. Make sure to start with the feelings about not having solved the problem or the decision not working out.

As noted previously, FIG TESPN can be implemented flexibly in a variety of settings. Despite the complexity of the skills involved, it is important to run through all the steps even if some are not given a full treatment. It is through the repetition that the process is mastered. Each time the process is repeated, a certain step or skill can be highlighted.

BRINGING FIG TESPN INTO THE SCHOOL

Probe

FIG TESPN can be implemented both formally through regularly scheduled classes and informally by school personnel as problems arise. The strategy "Probe" (see Table 4.2) is one way of implementing FIG TESPN in a spontaneous, informal manner. It can be taught to school personnel (and parents) through inservice training or consultation. It is highly recommended that Probe be taught in conjunction with the Guiding Principles discussed in Chapter 2 (see Table 2.1). In addition, have the person who is going to be using Probe role play several scenarios during training. Probe uses the FIG TESPN steps although it starts with the "I have a problem" step rather than "Feelings are my cue to problem solve" because knowing the problem and context will help the facilitator guide the ques-

---

TABLE 4.2. Probe

1. I WOULD LIKE TO KNOW EXACTLY WHAT HAPPENED. WHAT HAPPENED BEFORE THIS? WHAT WERE YOU DOING? WHAT WAS _____ DOING? WHAT HAPPENED AFTER? WHAT DID YOU DO THEN? (Encourage specifics and the sequence of events and actions.)

2. HOW ARE YOU FEELING? HOW ELSE ARE YOU FEELING? I NOTICE YOU SEEM _____. HOW DO YOU THINK _____ IS FEELING? (Be sure the child uses "feelings" words rather than descriptions of the problem or what he/she did. This is very difficult but important for the child to do.)

3. WHAT WOULD YOU LIKE TO HAVE HAPPEN? WHAT IS YOUR GOAL? (Have the child focus on what he/she wants. Remember not to direct the goal yourself. Also, make sure the child differentiates between a "goal" and something the child can do to achieve that goal.)

4. WHAT DID YOU TRY TO DO? WHAT HAVE YOU THOUGHT OF DOING? WHAT ELSE CAN YOU THINK OF DOING? (By asking what he/she already tried, you are making the child aware that this was an option he/she chose to use rather than an impulse or inevitable act. After this, have the child brainstorm as many things as possible. Do not critique at this point.)

5. WHAT MIGHT HAPPEN IF YOU _____? WHAT ELSE? (Review each option listed above and have the child anticipate the potential outcomes. Add outcomes that you are aware of but that the child may not have thought about.)

6. OF THE THINGS YOU THOUGHT ABOUT WHICH ONE SEEMS LIKE THE BEST THING TO TRY FIRST? (Remind the child of the goal and ask if this will enable him/her to achieve the goal.)

7. HOW WOULD YOU DO IT? WHAT IS YOUR PLAN? SHOW ME AND WE CAN PRACTICE. (Review who, what, where, and how. Anticipate problems in implementing the plan and how the child can deal with these. Through role playing, social skills can be taught that will enable the child to implement the plan successfully.)

8. WHAT IF THINGS DO NOT WORK OUT THE WAY YOU WANT? WHAT WOULD YOU DO THEN? WHAT ELSE COULD YOU TRY? (Prepare the child for potential frustration in achieving his/her goal. Have the child think about what he/she would do then, including repeating the FIG TESPN process. This step may need to be bypassed for younger children because it requires a greater level of cognitive sophistication.)

9. OKAY, THINK ABOUT IT, TRY IT, AND LET ME KNOW WHAT HAPPENS. (Have the child make a commitment to try the plan. Review with the child what he/she did or did not do. Do not get discouraged if the did not use the plan. Follow-up will be extremely important: it reinforces the child for problem solving, helps him/her adapt the plan as necessary, and lets him/her know you really care.)

tioning. If the situation is already known to the facilitator, then the first two steps can be reversed and the probing can start with how the individuals are feeling. Regardless of whether the problem is discussed first or second, it is important to elicit specific antecedents and consequences. When the child responds, "I don't know," use of the Columbo technique with patience and persistence will be particularly important.

FIG TESPN Intervention: Curriculum and Group Format

For maximum learning, it is helpful to schedule social problem-solving activities on a regular basis and to use a formal curriculum or structured, sequenced set of activities. *FIG TESPN Goes to Middle School* (Tobias, 1992) is an intervention guide that utilizes video to teach and practice the problem-solving steps. The curriculum consists of readiness skills activities and a series of FIG TESPN activities. After learning readiness skills and introduccing FIG TESPN, students watch videos and apply the problem-solving steps to the characters in the video.

The format (which applies to the activities described below) is as follows:

1. Review previous activities.
2. Share instances when students used previously taught skills.
3. Highlight a current skill to review and practice.
4. Run through the steps (FIG TESPN).
5. Introduce the videotape.
6. Play the videotape.
7. Discuss the videotape in the context of FIG TESPN with a focus on the highlighted skill.
8. Discuss application to real life.
9. Use auxiliary activities to reinforce the highlighted skill.

Although the curriculum was written based on the *Self-Incorporated* video series (Agency for Instructional Technology, 1994), any short video can be used. Commercially produced situation comedies are excellent resources. Without commercials, they run approximately 22 minutes, which leaves time for discussion in a 30- to 45-minute class. Although students do not like this, half the video can be shown in one class and completed in the following class if there are time constraints.

Situation comedies have the advantage of being popular with children and remaining current in terms of cultural mores. The programs follow a specific formula that will allow the facilitator to work FIG TESPN into the analysis of the program without preparation on the facilitator's part. However, the facilitator may wish to screen the program for appropriate content. For example, a particular concern is the prevalence of sexual references even in allegedly "family" shows. The "sitcom" formula is story set-up, problem/conflict presentation, and resolution. Most often, two story lines are presented. The class can focus on one or both. One story line can also be edited out or fast-forwarded. (More about the use of video and video resources can be found in Chapter 5.)

The following are several sample activity plans adapted from *FIG TESPN Goes to Middle School: An Intervention Guide* (Tobias, 1992).

ACTIVITY: INTRODUCTION TO "FIG TESPN"

Objectives

1. To introduce students to the steps of social decision making and problem solving.
2. To provide students with a centralizing concept so that the social decision-making and problem-solving steps can be remembered as a whole rather than as discrete steps.
3. To provide students and teachers with a prompt for problem solving.

Materials

Board, FIG TESPN handouts

Procedure

1. Review the readiness skills (Keep Calm, Be Your BEST, Feelings Fingerprints, Problem Trackers [see Tables 6.1 and 6.2]) and how students have used them.

2. Review what students have learned about feelings and how to deal with them. Review Feelings Fingerprints and how feelings are the cue to start problem solving.

3. Tell the students: "The purpose of today's activity is to introduce FIG TESPN but I am not really sure who or what FIG TESPN is. FIG TESPN helps you solve problems and helps you figure out how to do things in the best way possible. FIG helps you use your own resources and abilities rather than doing things for you. FIG helps you think before acting. FIG helps you decide the best thing to do to get what you want. FIG

comes on the scene when feelings become strong and people have difficulty deciding what to do." (FIG TESPN = Social Problem Solving.)

4. Generate from the students examples of who FIG TESPN might be like. If the students are having difficulty, discuss who provides guidance and helps others succeed without acting directly for them. If students cannot generate examples, suggest local or national sports coaches or managers and television or movie characters (Obi Wan Kenobe and Yoda from *Star Wars*, Jiminy Cricket from *Pinocchio*, Counselor Troi from *Star Trek: The Next Generation*). Stress that FIG TESPN does not solve the problem for the student or tell the student what to do; instead, FIG TESPN helps the student solve the problem.

5. Encourage students to develop their own image of who FIG TESPN is like. Have them discuss this with the class. Discourage students from using teachers or parents as their image; these persons are authority figures who often tell students what to do, whereas FIG TESPN helps students tell themselves what to do.

6. Distribute handouts of the FIG TESPN steps. Explain that FIG can help them solve problems by reminding them to ask themselves questions (e.g., "I have a problem" leads to "what is my problem?"). Have students read the steps and review relevant vocabulary and concepts.

7. Model a problem-solving situation using FIG's steps. Provide a semipersonal situation in which you solved a problem, made a decision, or had a conflict with someone.

8. Assign students to think about situations in which FIG TESPN's steps could be helpful to them. Review these situations at the beginning of the next activity.

Skill Builders

Note: It is important for students to be actively involved with FIG TESPN, to actually do something with it, in order to reinforce the concept and personalize it.

1. Have students draw pictures or computer-generated images of FIG TESPN.

2. Have students write stories about FIG TESPN. Topics include how FIG came to be, how FIG learned to be a good problem solver, why FIG likes to help others, how FIG helped solve someone's problem, and so forth.

3. Have a poster of FIG TESPN and the questions in the room for the students to refer to in subsequent activities and/or have them make their own copies of the steps and relevant questions. (See Tables 4.1 and 4.2.)

4. Have students draw a comic strip involving FIG TESPN.

5. Show the film *Pinocchio* or the recent television show *The Wonder Years* and discuss comparisons between FIG TESPN and Jiminy Cricket or between FIG and the voice that helps the main character think through his problems.

6. Give a writing assignment with a beginning (feeling and problem) and an end. Have the students fill in the middle of the story using FIG TESPN.

Tips for Teachers

1. Encourage students to be imaginative in their conception of FIG TESPN. Try to avoid priming them with preconceived images so as to ensure that students develop their own images. This will enhance use.

2. Avoid referring to FIG as "he" or "she" because FIG should be universal.

3. At a later time, FIG will become a prompt for problem solving. For example, "How could FIG help you with this?"

4. For older students, it may be best to deemphasize the use of FIG TESPN as a character and instead focus mainly on it as an acronym for remembering the steps of social decision making and problem solving, like SCUBA (self-contained underwater breathing apparatus).

5. Do not expect that students will completely understand or be able to use FIG TESPN after this brief introduction. Remember that FIG TESPN will be learned through repetition. Also, in subsequent activities, always do a complete run-through of FIG TESPN at least once in the activity.

6. Chapter 2 contains an extended example of how one can use FIG TESPN. In that dialog, a teacher is working with a class of students who already have been introduced to FIG TESPN. Note how the group leader, in this case a teacher, uses the techniques in Chapter 2, especially those in Table 2.1, to build the students' skills. (See pp. 28–31.)

ACTIVITY: FEELINGS CUE ME TO PROBLEM SOLVE

Objectives

1. To review the steps of social decision making and problem solving.
2. To reinforce the skill of identifying signs of different feelings.
3. To further understand and deal effectively with feelings.

Materials

Video equipment, Self-Incorporated videotape *Pressure Makes Perfect* (or other age-appropriate video)

Outline of Procedure (consistent for most subsequent activities)

1. Review previous activities.
2. Share instances when students used previously taught skills.
3. Highlight a current skill.
4. Run through the steps (FIG TESPN).
5. Introduce the videotape.
6. Play videotape.
7. Discuss the steps with a focus on the highlighted skill.
8. Discuss application to real life.

Procedure

1. Review assignment to think of problem situations in which FIG TESPN could help them out (Step 8 in Introduction Activity).

2. Review previous activities that dealt with feelings. Remind students that Keep Calm is a way of dealing with overwhelming feelings. Review Feelings Fingerprints and Trigger Situations.

3. Have students share with the class when they used Keep Calm or when they were aware of different feelings in others and how they knew what those feelings were.

4. Indicate that today's activity will help them practice identifying feelings a little more. Say: "The reason for this is that it can help you in real life. For example, if you want something from someone, it is usually helpful to be able to tell how they feel so that you'll ask them at a good time. Or, if sometimes you lose your temper and this has caused you problems, it is a good idea to be aware of your feelings so that you can control them."

5. Remind students that awareness of a feeling is the first step in problem solving. Remind students of FIG TESPN's steps. Have students read the steps out loud.

6. Run through the steps with the students. The teacher or the student can ask a question and then someone else can give a general response (i.e., not in reference to a specific problem).
For example:

Student: How am I feeling?

Other student: I feel angry.
Other student: I feel happy.
Student: What is the problem?
Other student: The problem is that someone is bothering me.

This can be done in a quick manner with the teacher pointing to a student and saying "question" (the student then says the next question in FIG TESPN, based on Table 4.2) and then pointing to another student who gives a feeling, problem, goal, option, and so forth.

7. Tell the students that they will be watching a videotape to help them practice identifying feelings and solving social problems. Say: "The first step in solving problems and making decisions is to notice signs of different feelings. They are the signal that there is a potential problem or that you might have to decide to do, or not do, something."

8. Review the plot of the video, which is about a girl who is practicing for a piano recital and is getting a lot of pressure from those around her. You may need to review some of the symbolism in the video (i.e., dream sequences, the bug, etc.).

Assign some students to look at body language—how the characters move their heads, hands, feet, and bodies. Others can look at facial expressions—what we see in faces. Others can listen to what the characters say and how their voices sound. Tell students that they may want to see if the characters are being their BEST.

9. Play all of the video.

10. At the end of the video, review what students were asked to look for. Make a chart of the following:

Who?   Had what feeling?   How could you tell?

Generate a list of situations and feelings.

11. Discuss one or more of the above situations in detail, introducing the FIG prompt to problem solve by saying something like, "How could FIG TESPN help the main character out?"

Say: "What's the first thing FIG reminds the girl to do [ask herself how she is feeling]? What should she do next?" and so forth. Be sure to go though all of the steps.

12. Encourage students to be aware of different feelings in themselves and others and how this may be helpful to them. Discuss several situations, such as the following:

+ You are talking to someone you want to impress and he/she looks bored.
+ You want to ask your parent if you can go out and he/she looks angry.
+ You want to be cool but sense yourself getting nervous.

13. Assign students to remember situations in which awareness of feelings, either their own or others', was helpful to them and have them share this with class during the next activity.

Tips for Teachers

1. Stress the importance of identifying feelings in others as well as in themselves. Students may find it easier to identify feelings in others than in themselves.

2. Introduce a flow chart. You may wish to have a permanent one in the room and use it for a new problem each week.

3. If you are using a videotape other than one from the Self-Incorporated series, be sure to review the tape prior to showing it to the class and give them a brief synopsis. The videotape should highlight and explore one or more feelings.

ACTIVITY: I HAVE A PROBLEM

Objectives

1. To have students identify interpersonal problems .
2. To review and reinforce the problem-solving steps.

Materials

Video equipment, Self-Incorporated videotape *Different Folks*

Outline of Procedure (see p. 62)

Procedure

1. Review previous activities that dealt with feelings. Remind students that Keep Calm is a way of dealing with overwhelming feelings. Review Feelings Fingerprints and Trigger Situations.

2. Have students share with the class when they used Keep Calm or when they were aware of different feelings in others and how they knew what those feelings were. Review assignment given on identifying different feelings (Step 13, Feelings Activity) and how this was helpful to them.

3. Indicate to the students that today's activity will focus on identifying problems and telling themselves what the problem is. Say: "Telling yourself the problem is the second step in problem solving."

4. Remind students of FIG TESPN steps. Run through the steps with the students by having one student ask a question and another give a response.

5. Tell the students that they will be watching a videotape to help them practice identifying and solving social problems.

Say: "The first step in solving problems and making decisions is to notice signs of different feelings. They are the signal that there is a potential problem or that you might have to decide to do, or not do, something.

"The second step is telling yourself what the problem is. Putting the problem into words and defining it can help you figure out what to do to solve it. This is because sometimes there are several problems and you need to work with them one at a time. Also, sometimes you may be confusing a feeling or a solution with a problem.

"For example, if you are walking through the hall and you are pushed into a locker, you may think that the problem is that you are angry and you want to punch the kid walking nearest to you. However, your feeling is one of anger but your problem may be that you need some way to express your anger, or your problem may be that some kids in school pick on you. Hitting the kid is only one possible option or solution to the problem, and not necessarily the best one in this situation.

"Another example is that you came to school angry because you forgot your homework. You can think about your feelings and then think about what exactly the problem is. The problem may be any of the following:

• You did your homework but left it home.
• You forgot to do your homework.
• You can't get detention this afternoon because you have to be somewhere after school.

"Put the problem into your own words and this will help you solve it. Each problem will have a different solution."

6. Say (if using the Self-Incorporated video; otherwise, modify): "In the video today, the main character, Matt, gets upset with his family situation. His mother is an animal doctor and makes most of the money for the family. His father works at home as an illustrator and does most of the housework. Doug, Matt's friend, and other kids tease him because Matt has to help with the housework. As we watch the video, we want to focus on how Matt is feeling and what the problem is."

7. Play all or part of the video.

8. At the end of the video, make a chart of:

Matt's feeling (anger, embarrassment)	How could you tell? (expression, voice)	Problem (kids were teasing)

You may wish to make a flow chart that includes all the steps.

9. Discuss one or more situations in detail by introducing the FIG TESPN prompt to problem solve by saying something like, "How could FIG TESPN help Matt out?" Prompt each problem-solving question and follow up until each response is clearly defined. For example, ask, "How is Matt feeling?" If the response is "bad," clarify what "bad" is. Then ask, "What next? What is the problem?" and so forth.

10. Have students be aware of different problems that they have during the week. Remind them that a feeling is sometimes the sign that there is a problem. Have them define problems in relation to classroom difficulties as they occur during the week.

11. Have students complete and discuss the "Problem Inventory" (Elias et al., 1992). (See Table 4.3.)

Tips for Teachers

At some point in the introduction of this step, it is necessary to point out that the step is called "I have a problem." Ownership of the problem is an extremely important aspect of this step. This entails taking responsibility not for creating the problem but for solving it.

For example, if a student got into a fight, the problem is not that another child started it (that is the other child's problem), but that the student is involved in it and needs to do something to resolve the conflict. Another example might be that the student failed a test; the problem is not that the test was too hard (which may be true) but that the student now has a failure for the marking period.

This focus on the student's ownership of the problem does not deny that others are involved but places responsibility for doing something about it on the student. In the example of the student failing the test because it was too hard, a potential solution is to talk to the teacher about it; however, the student has to initiate this interaction. The teacher does not have a problem; the student has the problem even though it might be the teacher's "fault." In the other example, the student who started the fight might be at "fault," but the student who was aggressed against has to do something about it.

This is a subtle concept that is not readily accepted by students. They often focus on blame and insist on the other person doing something. It is necessary for the teacher to refocus the student on what his/her part of the problem is and what he/she can do to solve it.

TABLE 4.3. Problem Inventory

Below is a list of things that might happen to you in middle school. Read each item. Circle the number 1, 2, 3, or 4 depending on how much of a problem it is for you. Use the following scale:

1 = This has not been a problem for me.
2 = This has been a small problem for me.
3 = This has been a medium-sized problem for me.
4 = This has been a large problem for me.

	Not a problem	Small problem	Medium problem	Large problem
1. Getting lost and not being able to find your way around school.	1	2	3	4
2. Forgetting your locker combination.	1	2	3	4
3. Being treated too much like a child.	1	2	3	4
4. Having school farther away from home.	1	2	3	4
5. Having a tough teacher.	1	2	3	4
6. Buying new notebooks.	1	2	3	4
7. Having harder work.	1	2	3	4
8. Eating in a larger cafeteria.	1	2	3	4
9. Having an argument with a teacher.	1	2	3	4
10. Being sent to the office.	1	2	3	4
11. Forgetting to bring the right books to class.	1	2	3	4
12. Getting too much homework.	1	2	3	4
13. Getting into fights.	1	2	3	4
14. Missing friends from elementary school.	1	2	3	4
15. Having trouble making new friends.	1	2	3	4
16. Wishing you were not in special classes.	1	2	3	4
17. Kids trying to talk you into something.	1	2	3	4
18. Getting things stolen from you.	1	2	3	4
19. Getting bothered by older kids.	1	2	3	4
20. Not getting along with all your different teachers.	1	2	3	4
21. Other kids teasing you.	1	2	3	4
22. Being left out of the popular group.	1	2	3	4
23. Changing in the locker room for gym class.	1	2	3	4
24. Drinking alcohol.	1	2	3	4
25. Getting involved with drugs.	1	2	3	4
26. Smoking cigarettes.	1	2	3	4
27. Dating girls/boys.	1	2	3	4
28. Teachers expecting too much of you.	1	2	3	4

ACTIVITY: THINK OF MANY POSSIBLE THINGS TO DO

Objectives

1. To have students generate behavioral alternatives for problem solving.
2. To review and reinforce the problem-solving steps.

Materials

Video equipment, Self-Incorporated videotape *By Whose Rules?*

Outline of Procedure (see p. 62)

Procedure

1. Review the previous activity, [which would have dealt with goal setting in the full curriculum], and any homework assignments relative to identifying and setting goals.

2. Generate testimonials from students as to when they used previous skills (Keep Calm, Be Your BEST) or were aware of situations in which they could have used FIG TESPN.

3. Tell students that today's activity will focus on generating options. Have students define what an "option" is. Indicate that this is the next step in problem solving after identifying goals.

4. Say: "In order to reach a goal, you must actually do something. Although you might not realize it at first, there are always different ways to reach the goal and different things that you can do. The hard part is being aware of all the different things that you could do to reach your goal. The more possibilities you can think of, the more options you will have to chose from, and the easier it will be to reach your goal."

5. Say: "Before you actually start to think of options, it may be helpful first to Keep Calm. Remember, you will need to think of options when there is a problem and when feelings might be strong. Therefore, it might be helpful first to stop and calm yourself down. This will better enable you to think before you act and will give you a better chance of reaching your goal."

6. Say: "Thinking of options is sometimes called 'brainstorming.' This is used often in business when people are trying to come up with new ideas and new ways of doing things. Brainstorming involves people thinking of all the ideas that they can without first being critical of them. After

you think of them, then you go back and look at them a little more critically. We will do this in the next step, when we 'envision outcomes.'"

7. Practice brainstorming with the students. Use a typical problem that students have in class or ask a student to volunteer a problem or goal. With the example, briefly explore feelings and goals before generating options. Allow students to be creative in their options (within limits).

8. Remind students of FIG TESPN steps. Run through the steps with the students.

9. Tell the students that they will be watching a videotape to help them practice generating options.

10. Give an outline of the video.

11. Play all or part of the video.

12. After viewing the video, make a chart of:

Feeling   Problem   Goal   Options

13. Discuss one or more situations in detail by introducing the FIG prompt to problem solve. Follow through with all the problem-solving steps for at least one option.

14. Additional exercise: Give students the beginning and end of a story and have them fill in the middle—that is, what option the characters in the story used that led to the outcome of the story. Compare the different options that the different students chose. This can be a writing assignment or can be done orally. An example beginning and end might be: "John had a big game coming up next week and he needed to practice. Unfortunately, he also had a test in science, which he was in danger of failing, and his best friend had tickets to see a concert that week. In the end, John felt good that he was able to get his work done and practice, and also felt pretty good about how he had handled the situation with his friend."

Or, you can use a beginning and end from a story the students have read or are familiar with and have them generate different options for the characters.

ACTIVITY: ENVISION OUTCOMES

Objectives

1. To have students be aware of consequences.
2. To have students begin to anticipate the consequences of possible actions.
3. To review and reinforce the problem-solving steps.

Materials

Video equipment, Self-Incorporated videotape *Who Wins?*

Outline of Procedure (see p. 62)

Procedure

1. Review previous activities that dealt with goal setting and generating options.
2. Have students share examples of goals and options they had during the week. Review any homework assignments.
3. Generate testimonials from students as to when they used previous skills (Keep Calm, Be Your BEST) or were aware of situations in which they could have used FIG TESPN.
4. Tell students that today's activity will focus on envisioning the consequences or outcomes of various options that they have generated. Define key words, "envision," "consequence," and "outcome."
5. In order to teach students this skill, you will first teach them a visualization exercise. Students will not be expected to use this technique each time they are trying to make a decision but it is included as a means of encouraging students to anticipate consequences.

   a. Say: "We are now going to practice 'envisioning.' Although you probably won't do this in real-life problem situations that you are trying to solve, I think it will be fun and helpful for you to experience thinking ahead in a creative way."
   b. Say: "First, get comfortable in your seats and close your eyes. . . . Now, repeat the Keep Calm exercise to yourselves three times."
   c. Next describe a scene to the students and have them visualize the details. For example, say: "Imagine yourselves at a secluded beach. It's a hot, sunny day. You are lying there in the sun, relaxing. All of a sudden, an old, wooden sailing ship comes into view and a smaller boat with several men in it start rowing towards you. Think about what might happen next. I will ask you to open your eyes in a moment and tell us what you saw. . . . Okay, open your eyes."
   d. Discuss what the students saw.
   e. Another example, say: "You are in school, walking though the hall early in the morning. Someone bumps into you. You are really angry at them for knocking your books to the floor. You yell at them. What might happen next?"

6. Discuss with students why it is important to try to anticipate the consequences or outcomes of actions. Explain that for every action there is a consequence. Have students generate examples of actions and consequences.

7. Give students a problem situation, a goal, and several options. For example, "Someone is teasing you, you want him to stop teasing you. Your options are to beat him up, ignore him, tell the teacher, tell your parents, or never go to school again." Have the class generate possible consequences for each option. Draw a flow chart on the board with the options and consequences.

Beat him up _____

_____

_____

_____

Ignore him _____

_____

_____

_____

Tell on him _____

_____

_____

_____

Never go to school again _____

_____

_____

_____

8. Tell students that when thinking of consequences it is important to be creative and thorough. Also, every option has at least one possible consequence or outcome but it is important to think of as many as you can.

9. Introduce the video in which the students will have to think of options and consequences of those options at the end. Say (if using the Self-

Incorporated video): "This video is about two friends, Lenny and Brant, who are in competition with one another in a photography contest. Lenny's best picture gets ruined by Brant. Lenny has to decide what to do. You'll see what his options are and then we will discuss the potential consequences of those options."

10. Play the video.

11. After the video, make a flow chart like the one above and have the students fill in the possible consequences.

12. Use FIG TESPN to solve Lenny's problem.

13. An additional exercise for students might be to give them an unfinished story and have them make up various endings. This can be done as an individual writing assignment or as a group discussion.

ACTIVITY: NOTICE WHAT HAPPENED AND REMEMBER IT FOR NEXT TIME

Objectives

1. To teach students self-monitoring.
2. To emphasize follow-through.
3. To reinforce the steps of social decision making and problem solving.
4. To teach students that despite their best efforts, their plan might not be successful and they may have to rethink the problem, goal, or plan.

Materials

Students' plans from the previous activity

Procedure

1. Review students' FIG TESPNs with an emphasis on the plans.

2. Discuss with students the importance of following through with their plan. A plan is only as good as its implementation.

3. Ask students how their plans went. Did they end up doing what they said they would; if not, why not? Were there unanticipated obstacles? Did they get the reactions from others they expected? Did things go more easily than anticipated?

4. If a student did not carry out his plan, ask, "Why not?" Discuss what the obstacle to the plan was. The student may have been insufficiently motivated by the goal or lacked a necessary skill to implement the plan.

5. For those students whose plans did not succeed, do a "second-order" FIG TESPN. This involves taking the step at which the student got stuck and solving the problem around this obstacle. For example, a student may say that she was going to ask her father for an increase in allowance but did not have a chance. Guide the student through FIG TESPN around the problem that seemed to occur in the planning phase. How did she feel about not asking her father? What was the problem? (he was busy, she was intimidated, etc.) What is her goal? and so forth.

6. For those students who succeeded in reaching their goal, ask them how they feel now as compared to their initial feeling.

7. Finally, ask students what they learned from this and can remember the next time they have this or a similar problem. Ask them what they learned from each other's FIG TESPNs.

Tips for Teachers

1. At some point in this activity, emphasize to students that it is also important for them to tell themselves how they did. Give the students examples of self-reinforcing statements, such as "I did a good job," or self-coping statements, such as "Well, my plan didn't work this time, but I can always rethink the problem and try another option."

2. Have students be aware of the feelings that they have after problem solving. Positive feelings indicate that the problem was solved. Negative feelings are a cue to reengage in problem solving (this brings them back full circle to identifying feelings).

3. You may wish to draw a second-order FIG TESPN on the board. An illustration of how this would apply when one is "stuck" trying to find an appropriate goal would look like this:

F
I
G – F
   I
   G
   T
   E
   S
   P
   N

This of course can be extended to third- and fourth-order FIG TESPNs.

For example, a student having a problem went through FIG TESPN and his goal was to get a kid to leave him alone. He tried his plan, which was to ignore the pesky kid. However, that kid continued to bother him and the student did not reach his goal. It was helpful at this point to do the second-order FIG TESPN and have the student discuss first how he felt about trying to ignore the pest and then having it not work. The problem turned out to be that the student had too little influence over whether or not the solution could work. Therefore, the student thought of other possible things to do that would address this issue, such as making friends with the kid, avoiding him altogether, and telling the principal. This was done in a brainstorming process, similar to when the student originally tried to "think of things to do." The student then proceeded with the rest of FIG TESPN, based on these new ideas, and eventually came up with a plan that led to the goal.

APPLICATION OF FIG TESPN TO EVERYDAY
INTERPERSONAL SITUATIONS

FIG TESPN can be applied to everyday problems encountered by students. Guided questioning by the teacher can facilitate resolution of peer conflicts, address persistent problems, and alleviate the anxiety generated by potential problems in the future by using FIG TESPN to develop a plan for students to cope with them.

If students are not getting along or there is a crisis situation, students can be taken aside together or individually and guided through the FIG TESPN steps with the use of Probe. It is important for the school practitioner working with students to function as facilitator rather than problem solver; in other words, the teacher does not tell the student what he or she should do, but rather helps the student focus on how to solve the problem by thinking through all aspects of it carefully. Students who are in a highly aroused emotional state will be resistant to discussing anything in a positive manner. It may be necessary to help them Keep Calm and practice BEST. It may also be helpful to have them write down what happened. This will give them time for the intensity of their emotions to abate and will introduce the cognitive component to solving their problem, which will reduce impulsivity.

Low-level, everyday, persistent problems can be addressed using FIG TESPN. For example, a student may be coming to class late every day. Such vexing annoyances as this distract from instructional time and impede positive classroom momentum. Teachers can be helped to indicate to the student that this is a problem that needs to be solved. In this instance, the teacher may indicate his or her feelings, problem, and goal and require the student to generate options for solving it. The teacher may include certain incentives as part of the plan; for example, coming to class on time every day for a week earns one less assignment and coming to class late 2 days in a row earns a detention. Forgetting homework, disruptions in class, and other common problems can also be dealt with. The teacher may facilitate problem solving and at times offer suggestions, but it is important to keep in mind that the more the student engages in the problem-solving process, the higher the chance for success. Teacher-implemented solutions rarely have the desired effect and do not teach the student how to solve problems independently.

Students also encounter many stresses in school that can be alleviated by FIG TESPN during a group sharing time. After FIG TESPN is taught, common issues can be brought up and discussed on a regular basis using FIG TESPN as a general discussion format (see the Problem Inventory in Table 4.3 for examples). The issues can either be presented by the facilitator or students. Problem Trackers (see Tables 6.1 and 6.2) are another source of sharing troublesome issues that can be shared by the class.

For example, FIG TESPN can help students organize and plan for studying for a test. FIG TESPN can prepare students for a transition to a new grade or school. FIG TESPN can also help students cope with potential social stresses such as trying out for a sports team or making new friends.

Chapter 6 discusses everyday applications with particular emphasis on discipline and guidance, and Chapter 7 gives examples of how FIG TESPN can be infused into diverse academic areas.

CHAPTER 5

♦♦♦

Flexible Video-Based Group Applications for High-Risk Youth

♦

In nearly two decades of work in dozens of school districts, with both public and private schools, the participants in the ISA-SPS Project (Elias & Clabby, 1989) have found an instructional technique called TVDRP to be highly effective with all groups of students. "TVDRP" refers to Television (or other audiovisual media), Discussion conducted with open-ended questions designed to stimulate critical thinking, and Rehearsal and guided Practice, often involving role play or other experiential, hands-on activities to make learning more concrete and promote integration and generalization. Researchers have found that the combination of all three modalities considerably exceeds any two of the approaches together (Salomon, 1979). Our experience in using TVDRP with diverse groups of children from early elementary through high school age, including children with severe emotional disturbance and learning impairments, reflects this as well.

The mechanism by which TVDRP works appears to reflect the following:

- ♦ The value of television as a means of focusing attention and exercising a calming and relaxing effect, even among children with neurological impairments or attention deficits.
- ♦ The stimulation of thinking and problem solving engendered by discussions built on open-ended questions and "dialoging."
- ♦ The motoric and interpersonal benefit of rehearsal, guided practice, and role play in solidifying behavior sequences and making transfer and generalization outside the instructional setting more likely (Elias, 1982; Salomon, 1979).

TVDRP emphasizes skill building in three critical areas: self-control, group participation and social awareness, and social problem solving. The last area, which is important to children's successful functioning in the social and academic mainstream, is taught by ensuring that discussions follow a common format across all television programs and all content areas. The format elicits thoughtful decision making and problem solving via guided questioning, of the kind described in Chapter 2. The inductive learning accomplished by repeated application of the Probe questioning strategy within the TVDRP framework has been demonstrated even in populations of inner-city youth from diverse multicultural backgrounds who have emotional and neurological impairments sufficiently serious to warrant their being placed in residential treatment (Elias, 1983).

THE VIDEO/TVDRP WORKSHEET/ACTIVITY GUIDE

Table 5.1 contains an outline of what can be used as a worksheet for students or as a guide to planning and carrying out TVDRP-related activities. The discussion typically begins with a review of the video shown. Here, students exercise their skills of memory and sequencing. Differences in recollection can be settled by going back to the video. Students learn the importance of "keeping straight" what they see and hear, and this activity provides a naturalistic opportunity to give them ways to sharpen those skills. Next, focal characters are selected and feelings are emphasized. Here, and at any point along the way, supplemental activities can be added to provide extra practice in areas in which students need to strengthen their skills. (See Cartledge & Milburn, 1984; Elias & Clabby, 1989, for specific activities.)

The discussion is guided through setting goals, brainstorming alternative solutions, considering positive and negative consequences, selecting an action that will help reach positive goals, planning the details of carrying out an action, and anticipating obstacles. Children derive much additional benefit from TVDRP when guided practice, rehearsal, and role plays with feedback are used to make discussions of plans and obstacles realistic and more likely to transfer to the real world.

To begin rehearsal and guided practice, teachers set the stage by describing the scene and characters and assigning roles to students. These students then act out the discussion, showing how they would carry out the plans. Other students are asked to provide obstacles (e.g., saying that a desired club is filled or that some supplies a student asked for are not available). The rest of the class has an important role in giving feedback about the ideas tried out and aspects of the presentation, such as the BEST skills—body posture, eye contact, the saying of appropriate words, and

TABLE 5.1. Outline of the Video Worksheet

1. Briefly summarize the story/video. What was it about?
2. Who are the main characters?
3. Choose one of the main characters. Say what that person's problem is, using one sentence.
4. Characters express their feelings in many ways, sometimes in words and sometimes by their tone of voice or the way their body or face looks. List the feelings expressed by the main character you chose.
5. When the characters express upset or uncomfortable or unpleasant feelings, it is their way of telling us they want to find a way to solve a problem of some kind. What is your character's goal? What would he or she like to have happen?
6. To get ready to solve a problem or make a decision, it is helpful to envision or picture in your mind many different ways to get to a goal. This is called brainstorming ideas. We can practice brainstorming like this: [Show a picture of an abstract shape, such as one of the following:]

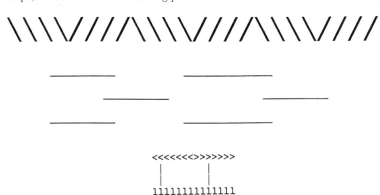

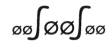

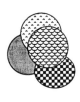

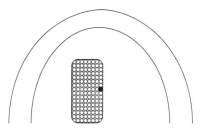

What could this picture be? Write down as many ideas as you can. Have fun!

7. Share your ideas with your group/class. Some of your ideas may be the same as others', and some might be different. How many *different* ideas did your group/class discover?

8. Look back at steps 3, 4, and 5. You picked a main character, and that character has a problem to solve. On your own, write down *as many ways* to reach the goal as you can think of.

9. How many ideas did you think of? _____ Share your ideas with your group or class. How many *different* ideas did your group or class come up with? On a separate piece of paper or on the board, write all of these ideas into a single big list.

10. A good idea is an idea that helps solve a problem and reach a goal without hurting anybody. For each idea on the big list, envision, or picture in your mind, whether or not it is a good idea. Put a "+" next to each one that you think is a good idea, and put a "–" next to each one that you think is not a good idea. If you are not sure about an idea, put a "?" next to it.

11. Make a new list of the best ideas. This list will include all the ones with a "+" next to them. Also, take another look at the ones marked with a "?" and see if any of them might be an idea you would try if you had a problem like the one in the video or story.

12. Be sure that everyone in the group or class shares the list of best ideas. Be sure to get the group or class to decide on one, two, or even three of the best ideas.

13. Next, plan how each of the solutions will be carried out. When will it happen? Where? What words will be said? How? Who needs to be there? Take turns trying out the plan and giving each other feedback until it seems to be the best plan.

14. Envision any roadblocks that might get in the way of your plan. What might go wrong? Can you learn from what happened to you or anyone else when you tried the same kinds of solution and action plan? How would you change your plans to get around the roadblocks?

15. Return to the video and choose another character and problem. Work it through on a new worksheet. Also, you may try the same process with problems from another video.

voice tone. Scenes usually are played again—sometimes to give members of the student audience a turn at center stage. Throughout, teachers are director/coaches and should feel free to help the actors portray the roles even as the action is occurring. Active coaching provides students with feedback and support and maximizes their learning. (For detailed guidelines on carrying out guided practice and role plays, see Cartledge & Milburn, 1980; Elias & Clabby, 1989.)

The whole worksheet/TVDRP process, which spans at least several class periods, can be repeated for another segment of a video, another character in a video, or another video. Discussion can be held with or without use of a worksheet. Similarly, the worksheet can include all or part of what is presented. We have been successful with cooperative learning and small group or full-class formats in both self-contained classes for children with disabilities and mainstream classes. Videos can be selected from the fine series available from public television, such as *Inside/Out*, *Thinkabout*, *On the Level*, at elementary, middle school, and high school levels; former television shows, such as *The Wonder Years*, *DeGrassi High* and *DeGrassi Junior High*, and *The Cosby Show*; episodes from various *Star Trek* series; video series such as *Roots* and *Eyes on the Prize*, and movies such as *An American Tail*, *The Sword and the Stone*, *Roxanne*, and *Glory*.

Making It Work

In our experience, with appropriate materials, even elementary school children and those with behavioral and attentional problems have been able to manage video segments of up to 15 minutes and follow-up discussions of 10 to 15 minutes (Elias, 1983). However, many factors might influence these time estimates. It might be necessary to begin with shorter segments until it is clear that students are able to handle more, which can be expected with practice. A given video segment can serve as the material of many lessons, especially as supplemental skill-building activities are incorporated. Where students with special behavioral or learning needs are involved, lessons should be held two to three times per week to sustain continuity. After some practice with video-based activities, students may be sufficiently comfortable and prepared to respond to questions such as, "What about a time when you have had problems like the one we saw in the video? What might you be feeling?" and "What would you want to have happen?" Teachers and other group leaders should begin with the discussion guide format and then make changes to fit their particular populations and needs. Exchanging ideas with other teachers using TVDRP instructions is another valuable way to build a repertoire of TVDRP strategies.

THE VIDEO CRITIQUE CLUB

There are some students and some contexts for which an alternative approach to TVDRP is most effective. The Video Critique Club is a concept that capitalizes on some students' tendencies to be oppositional or disinterested in just about anything introduced by an adult or an authority figure. It also is useful when one is working with a heterogeneous group and can guarantee that a significant minority of the class will not be able to, or wish to, identify with the age, ethnicity, gender, or "coolness" of a video's protagonist(s). The club format is additionally useful in that one can form a "clinical" group but avoid the stigma and negative labeling involved. The rationale for a club is a chance to get together and do something interesting related to television and videos. One presents students with an opportunity to be like their favorite movie critics, whether Siskel and Ebert, Lyons and Medved, or the reviewers on MTV. They are told that they will meet for a given number of weeks (at least 4, and as long as one, two, three, or four marking periods) and they will review videos. This tends to produce some level of positive motivation in even oppositional and disaffected students.

The skill development aspect of the critique approach comes in several ways. First of all, students share their views about the videos, which helps build their accuracy in processing cues in the environment. When students disagree about whether something was or was not said or shown, the group leader need only "go to the videotape" and allow students to resolve the issue largely on their own. Second, the main skill learning comes in the group interaction. Here, the leader plays an important role in helping students to use Keep Calm and to use the BEST skills with one another. Further, brainstorming, envisioning consequences, planning, and anticipating obstacles are prominent aspects of the group tasks, thus giving the group leader many opportunities to use FIG TESPN and the Guiding Principles (see Chapter 2) to promote students' critical thinking, perspective taking, and interpersonal skill development. Yet, all this is done in the service of helping the groups complete tasks they are interested in completing, not simply as part of a "clinical" or "special education" or related "official" agenda.

When they meet, the framework in Table 5.2 is used to guide the meeting. At first, the group leader selects the videos. There is no need to be defensive about them; it is fine if the students adopt a critical attitude toward them. After clarifying the purpose of the video, the next step is to get a general rating, using the Popcorn Box rating system. At this point, or shortly thereafter, it is advisable to have students work in subgroups of four or five. How one groups them depends on one's larger purposes (e.g.,

TABLE 5.2. Outline of the Video Critique Club

1. Name of the critic: _____

2. Name of the video: _____

3. Date watched: _____

4. What is the goal of this video? Why is it supposed to be worth watching?

5. How much did you like the video?

   a. a lot   b. it was okay   c. a little   d. not at all

6. Popcorn Box rating system:

   On a scale of 1–5 boxes of popcorn, with 1 box being the worst and 5 boxes being the best, how many boxes of popcorn would you give it?

	1	2	3	4	5

7. What parts did you like the best?

8. What parts did you like the least?

9. Look at the parts you liked the best. With your group, discuss why you felt that way. Then, look at the parts you like the least. Again, discuss with your group why you felt that way. Then, agree as a group on the three parts that your group would most like to change. Write them below.

10. Next, together with your group, pick one of these parts to work on. Write it down, and then discuss and write down three different ways to improve upon the part you liked the least. (It is fine to combine two or three parts you liked the least and work on them together, if it makes sense to do so.)

11. With your group, discuss your ideas and plan a script change. Remember how much time you have to work with, both in terms of the video segment you are working on and the time you have to work on this critique. Be sure to picture in your mind the goal of the video, who will see it, and everything that will go into changing the video.

12. Rehearse your changes and improve your script. If possible, make an audio or video of your changes. If there is time, go back and work on changing other parts that you liked least. Share your changes with other groups and get and give feedback.

---

by gender; to mix genders; to mix students of different racial, ethnic, and/or socioeconomic groups; to mix academic levels; to foster mainstreaming or inclusion).

As one asks the questions in the framework, the students are being moved to be critical thinkers and reporters about what they have observed. They also must arrive at consensus on some points, which exercises many of the readiness skills, especially listening to others, taking others' perspective, keeping calm, and giving and receiving praise, help, and criticism. Moreover, they are challenged in questions 5 and 6 first to be constructive about what they have seen and then, and only then, to point out areas they disliked.

The essence of the procedure is to move the children to identify clearly what they dislike and then become engaged in doing something about it. That is shown in questions 7 and 8, where children are asked to indicate how they would change that which they did not like.

The next stage is perhaps the most educational: The students work in small groups to create their alternative versions. This will provide a venue to observe and give feedback on their interpersonal styles, especially the attributes described in BEST. Here, rather than didactically instructing students, skill development occurs in the context of in vivo examples, in situations in which students are motivated to get along because they are interested in completing the project. Indeed, to provide extra motivation for the project, one can offer to audio- or videotape the students' changes, have other subgroups give feedback, and further modify the alternative version.

An additional option for adolescents is to show them public service announcements related to prevention of such problems as alcohol, tobacco, steroid, or other drug use; HIV/AIDS; teenage pregnancy; violence, or guns, in schools; citizenship and voting; staying in school; or related themes. The video critique method can be used here, and the revised public service spots can be shown at an assembly, presented to the other schools, shown to (and perhaps created for) children in younger grades, or presented to the Board of Education, Town Council or other local government body, or even for a local business roundtable as part of a prevention fund raiser, such as for an alcohol-free senior prom night.

An initial choice is what type of video to bring in first. One useful strategy is to convene the groups of prospective critics and give them options: a television show, a movie-length video, or a public service announcement. Of course, the context in which the group is meeting also may constrain the choices students can be given. For example, if the club, or the critique concept, is being used as part of a health class, then the videos must relate to some aspect of health that is part of the curriculum. Here, the public service announcements often are the source of much learning. The videos themselves are short, and it is more feasible for students to create their own versions of these than it would be to work with movie-length material.

One other logistical point relates to preparation. Because students who are oppositional and lack motivation tend not to be interested in the preparatory activities, we have found it a useful strategy just to show the video, and then go back and elaborate the issues, along with a more careful reviewing of the video. Beginning with the videos serves as a gateway into the activities, taking advantage of the attention-getting aspects of the TVDRP approach. Among the movies that work well for the club at the high school level are *Schindler's List, Boyz 'N the Hood, Platoon,* and *Philadel-*

phia. At the middle school level, *Searching for Bobby Fischer, Angels in the Out-field,* and *It's a Wonderful Life* deal with themes related to family life, parent–child relationships, the importance of community, and related areas that might be important for certain groups of students to think about and act upon. One must leave ample time for TVDRP-based activities, especially those that involve creating products. With age-appropriate material chosen, those working with the Club can expect powerful discussions and projects.

GROUPS BASED ON MAKING COMMERCIALS, PUBLIC SERVICE SPOTS, AND DOCUMENTARIES

Rubinstein (1993) has created the "Social Decision Making Video Curriculum," an approach to TVDRP-based intervention that is of particular appeal to high-risk, disaffected, poorly motivated, and other special needs youth at the secondary school level. The "Mini-Unit on Advertising and Commercials" uses the FIG TESPN framework to help students learn about how advertisers sell products and to see video or television productions from the perspective of a critic, or of the person making the video. Different lessons help students learn to analyze the media, to understand the feelings that commercials and ads induce in viewers, to notice advertising appeals, and to create scripts, including the use of storyboards. A group based on the Mini-Unit could take approximately eight sessions, but

---

TABLE 5.3. Outline of a Social Problem-Solving Approach to Viewing Commercials

1. Type of product: _____

2. Name of product: _____

3. To whom does the product appeal?

4. What advertising appeals did you notice in the commercials?

5. What feelings did you experience while viewing the commercial?

6. Would you consider buying this product?

7. If you were remaking the commercial, what would you do differently? Some questions you may consider asking are:
   a. Is the name of the product a catchy one? Do you remember it easily?
   b. Would you choose to appeal to a different group of buyers? Why or why not?
   c. Think of alternative advertising appeals you might choose. What would be the consequences of those choices?

Note: This format can be adapted to radio or print advertising, as well as to a focus on public service messages and in-school or in-district publicity efforts.

could easily be extended by creating different types of commercials. Table 5.3 contains an outline of the procedure for viewing commercials.

Other resources in the video curriculum include modules on how to create documentaries and how to videotape students as they practice social decision-making skills (Rubinstein, 1993). The latter has special use for children who would benefit from feedback concerning their social skills performance. The former has been used in the context of academic subject areas, such as social studies, history, environmental science, community service, health, family life education, and high school courses such as psychology, justice, and vocational education. In the context of special education, students have derived considerable benefit from doing documentaries on their own handicapping conditions, with the attendant research and interviewing involved.

TALKING WITH TJ

An outstanding video resource available to those working with students at the elementary school level is the *Talking with TJ* series. The series is a short-term video-based program for use om afterschool child care, youth clubs and organizations, and the elementary grades. The program is best used by children in grades 2–4, although extensions upward and downward by one grade have been found to work. Developed under the auspices of the Hallmark Corporate Foundation (1994), with Dr. Karen Bartz as project manager, the TJ program initially was designed for use by youth leaders in youth organizations such as the Boys and Girls Clubs of America, 4-H Youth Development Education, and Girl Scouts of America; the latter organizations actually participated in the development, pilot testing, and initial field dissemination of the program. In addition, a team of scientific advisers in the areas of media, child development, preventive intervention, and multicultural education, evaluation experts at the University of Michigan, RMC Research Corporation, Arizona State University, University of Cincinnati, and Interwest Applied Research, innovative curriculum developers based at the University of Minnesota; and television production geniuses based at Paramount and VU productions all participated in a multiyear program development and evaluation process involving hundreds of thousands of adults as group leaders and literally millions of children as program recipients. As of this writing, the first two of three phases of the TJ program have been completed.

The TJ program has now been made available for use in schools, and it represents an outstanding resource for TVDRP-based, social problem-solving oriented interventions led by school practitioners. *Talking with TJ* is formulated as an effort to promote needed social competencies and interpersonal skills in young children, and as a primary prevention program for youth violence. It incorporates both the readiness skills and the use of problem solving as key components, and its design follows both the TV-DRP approach and the framework of "How to Develop a Skill" presented on pages 32–35 and Table 2.2.

The first phase of the project led to the production of a series focusing on the importance of cooperation and teamwork. Skills in the following three areas are emphasized:

1. Making group plans
2. Appreciating differences, and including people of diverse backgrounds in group activities as opportunities for learning, not situations to be avoided or feared
3. Playing as a cooperative team in competitive situations.

The basic program is structured around two sessions devoted to each of the three skill areas. A video is linked to each of the skill areas ("What's the Plan?" "All Together Now!" and "Team Spirit") and is designed with a TVDRP format. The first of the two sessions on each skill features an introductory discussion, a 15-minute video story, discussion, and short experiential activities. The second session involves a review of the video and a longer set of activities. One or more additional sessions can be devoted to the same skill, either by replaying and focusing on different aspects of the video and/or by expanding the provided activities or including additional ones. A concluding session consists of a "TJ Celebrate!" party.

Each of the videos shows a group of children solving a problem with the guidance of an engaging, energetic, young radio talk-show host named TJ the DJ. TJ and her helpers—teenager Jeff, who is her engineer, and Ray Dio, a veteran DJ who owns the station—both model and facilitate the use of self-calming and problem-solving techniques. Skills are reinforced through "power phrases" that are part of the discussion that surrounds each of the videos. There is "Talk Time" midway through the video, as well as discussion afterward that allows kids to relate the video to things that have happened in their lives. Other aspects of the instructional package include take-home information, in the form of a minicomic summarizing the video story; a home activity to reinforce program goals; and a how-to guide for group leaders including a detailed modeling video and specific directions for carrying out sessions, promoting the program, adapting sessions for special needs, and linking the skills into ongoing programs and activities in the setting. Carry-over activities include forming a "TJ Club" (in which the children give advice and help others solve problems or carry out team tasks cooperatively) or creating their own new TJ video or role-played episodes, focusing on building prosocial skills.

The second series focuses on conflict resolution and violence prevention and is called, *Talking with TJ about Working It Out*. The format is similar to the Teamwork series, except that for each video, there is a 5-minute recap video to be shown at subsequent meetings—especially useful for catching up absentees—and the training video included as part of the TJ Kit is more extensive. The focal skills are as follows:

1. Understanding feelings of anger, the consequences of violence, and different ways to respond when dealing with anger
2. Understanding different perspectives and working out win–win solutions
3. Learning how to use friendly phrases instead of fighting phrases, to diffuse anger and promote good communication

Evaluation results to date have found genuine enthusiasm for the program on the part of implementers and children. Children appeared to have learned the basic themes of each sessions, and responded well to transfer scenarios designed to test for generalization of skills from the TJ program to new problem situations. Children stated their intention to use "TJ behaviors" in their lives, and over 50% of all leaders reported explicit examples of seeing children use TJ behaviors in group sessions subsequent to TJ lessons. The latter survey took place 1–2 months after the sessions (Johnston, Bauman, Milne, & Urdan, 1993).

School practitioners will find TJ is superb for general classroom use, for clubs or targeted short-term groups for designated children, and an invaluable technique to provide structure and a positive, prosocial framework into afterschool child-care settings (Epstein, Elias, & Lefkowitz, 1995).

CONCLUSION

All children need skills to handle the demands of everyday living and of being a productive citizen in a democracy. Approaching school work and interpersonal decisions and problems in a thoughtful manner clearly is a desirable skill for all children, including those with disabilities, and such skills can be developed explicitly. The TVDRP technique and the various video and discussion guides, outlines, and activities presented can make important contributions toward that end (Mirman et al., 1988).

CHAPTER 6

Interventions into the
Discipline Sytem

♦

An effort to treat children with respect is likely to result in the
creation of opportunities for them to talk, reason (with authority),
and consider the long-term consequences of their actions and
make explicit and discuss the values, codes, and long-term
considerations that should guide those actions. In the course of
doing this, children will practice complex cognitive activities.
They will, for example, imagine and anticipate possible long-term
consequences of their actions. They will imagine barriers to
achieving their goals. They will consider a broad range of
possibly conflicting consequences of their actions and choose
between them. They will develop confidence in their ability to
handle ideas, come to think of themselves as individuals capable
of handling such ideas, and who have a right to opinions of their
own. They will come to think of authority as something that is
open to reason.

—Raven (1987, pp. 31–32)

The fundamental question each school and each classroom must address,
Sarason (1990) notes, is, "How should we live together and why?" The discipline procedures of a school and classroom are statements of its "constitution," its values, its essential beliefs about how people are to interact. A
discipline system is more than a vehicle to manage persistent or severe behavior problems. It is an expression of humanity, and, as such, can benefit
from a constructive problem-solving approach.

Behavioral problems such as frequent and severe disciplinary actions
(expulsions or suspensions) (Orr, 1987) and problems dealing with teachers

and other authority figures (Bhaerman & Kopp, 1988; Orr, 1987; Wells, 1990) do not only reflect individual children having difficulty. They are disruptive forces in a classroom or school and erode the sense of connection and community that is so important to learning (Hechinger, 1992). The Panel on High Risk Youth of the National Research Council (1993), in reviewing the literature on how to handle adolescents with aggressive, violent, and antisocial behavior, stated unequivocally that punitive approaches are singularly unsuccessful in creating positive behavior change or greater attention to negative consequences. Such approaches are more likely to breed resentment and revenge than contrition, and to set up cycles of accelerated misbehavior, punishment, and retribution—until the offending person is removed from the setting, more for social control reasons than for any likelihood of rehabilitation.

Attendance and discipline problems often are linked to academic difficulties and peer and familial stressors, and signal the start of a cyclical process that places many students on a path of increasing alienation from school (Bhaerman & Kopp, 1988; Brendtro et al., 1991; Elias et al., 1992). Beginning in middle school, intense discipline problems often are handled by suspending students from school—which communicates a lack of belonging and acceptance. Coupled with little support from school personnel, students become increasingly pessimistic about the possibility of school success, which further fuels their disinterest and feelings of alienation in school. They are uninvolved in school activities and do not identify with school values (Bhaerman & Kopp, 1988; Wells, 1990). They tend to be isolated within school and their main social outlets likely are friends who feel similarly; under such circumstances, the potential for angry (violent) or self-destructive (substance use, suicide, dropout) behavior is considerable (Bhaerman & Kopp, 1988; Wells, 1990).

There are reciprocal relationships between student characteristics and school processes leading to dropping out or "drifting out" (Natriello, Pallas, & McDill, 1986; Natriello, Pallas, McDill, McPortland, & Royster, 1988). Special education students in the secondary school environment often feel rejected by the school and experience what is referred to as being "pushed out" (Mahood, 1981; Natriello, Pallas, McDill, McPortland, & Royster, 1988). Regardless of educational classification, those who drop out prior to completing high school are at an enormous disadvantage in terms of economic opportunity and social and health status; they are more likely to find themselves in need of public financial assistance, or residing in correctional facilities (Burch, 1992). This disadvantage is significantly greater for members of minority groups, especially Latinos and African-Americans (Burch, 1992).

One of the maintaining factors in negative behavior patterns is impulsive decision making, which often leads to substance abuse, delinquent behavior, teen pregnancy, and parasuicidal behavior (Bhaerman & Kopp, 1988). Poor decision making also has been related to students' low self-esteem, feelings of powerlessness, low aspirations, and poor overall mental and physical well-being. Interventions with special education students based on teaching them interpersonal problem-solving skills have generally been successful, according to two recent reviews (Ager & Cole, 1991; Zaragoza, Vaughn, & McIntosh, 1991). Studies have shown that helping children develop a problem-solving strategy and combining it with opportunities to practice it and obtain feedback are especially effective with special needs populations (McIntosh, Vaughn, & Zaragoza, 1991; Small & Schinke, 1983). Lickona (1991) reports that using this kind of disciplinary inquiry technique not only decreases students' negative behavior, but it also increases students' sense of responsibility. The most critical factor promoting generalization of skills appears to be students' development of their metacognitive abilities; that is, they need to monitor their own thinking in interpersonal situations and consciously invoke a strategy and apply it (Mirman et al., 1988; Palincsar & Brown, 1985).

THE PROBLEM TRACKER: A TOOL FOR USE IN GROUP GUIDANCE, CLASS SHARING, OR LIFE SKILLS INSTRUCTION

A common element in group guidance, class sharing, and life skills instruction is to have students keep track of concerns, problems, or difficulties they encounter and bring them to the group for sharing and discussion. To make it more likely that students actually keep track of problems and to provide a consistent framework for thinking through these problems in a way that builds students' social decision-making skills, educators can use a "Problem Tracker" (Tables 6.1 and 6.2). The Problem Tracker is based on the Problem Diary (Elias & Clabby, 1989), a technique for self-monitoring how well one handles stressful situations. The Problem Tracker outline can be modified to become a worksheet that can allow students of any grade to write or depict situations that they would like to bring to the attention of their group (or just to the instructor).

The format in Table 6.2 was developed to minimize writing demands for those children with written language deficits or phobia. One certainly could make other modifications to tailor the Problem Tracker to the needs of particular populations being worked with. For example, specific Trigger Situations could be listed, as could a feelings vocabulary with which students might be familiar.

The formats use an inductive, self-questioning procedure to help students think through their concerns or problems and move toward appro-

TABLE 6.1. The Problem Tracker

Name: _____

Date: _____

1. In this space, write (or draw) what it is that is bothering you or that was a problem for you this week. Try to include *who* is involved and *when* or *where* it is taking place.

2. What did you say and do? *or* What would you like to say and do?

3. What happened in the end? *or* What would you like to have happen?

4. So far, how easy or hard has it been for you to stay calm and under control when dealing with this? (circle one number)

1	2	3	4	5
Very easy to control myself	Pretty easy	So-so	Pretty hard	Very hard to control myself

5. How satisfied are you with how you have been trying to solve the problem so far?

1	2	3	4	5
Not at all	Only a little	So-so	Pretty satisfied	Very, very satisfied

6. What do you like about what you have been doing so far?

7. What don't you like about what you have been doing so far?

8. What are some other ways you can handle the situation?

---

priate action. Teachers (and principals) of regular and special education students have found it useful to have a Problem Tracker handy and direct students to fill it out when they are upset or troubled *before* talking to adults about the situation or what they have done. Having students fill out the Tracker (or dictating one's responses, if necessary) provides a buffer that allows for more thoughtful discussion. It also makes it clear that students are responsible for trying to solve their problems.

RAPS Groups

One school psychologist with whom we have worked used the Problem Tracker to conduct groups in the high school that we have come to refer to as "RAPS groups," with RAPS standing for Repeated Applications of Problem Solving. The procedure was simple: Students all would have access to Problem Trackers, and during the week, they would fill them out and bring them to the group or drop them off with the school psychologist so that he could bring up the problem to the group in an anonymous way. The group would discuss the problem and spend the bulk of the time on

TABLE 6.2. The Problem Tracker

Name:_____ Date:_____ A.M. P.M.

1. Where were you? (Circle where the trouble happened.)

Classroom	School bus	Neighborhood
Hallway	Music or art	Friend's house
Lunchroom	Home	Gym
On the way to or from school		Other:_____

2. What happened? (Circle what happened.)

Somebody teased me.	Somebody called me a name.
Somebody took something of mine.	I did something wrong.
Somebody told me to do something.	Somebody started to fight.

   Other:_____

3. Who was that somebody? _____

4. How did you feel? (Circle how you felt.)

Embarrassed	Angry	Hurt	Guilty
Ashamed	Jealous	Happy	Surprised
Sad	Upset	Other:_____	

5. How could you tell? Circle your Feelings Fingerprints.

Head	Muscles	Stomach	Skin	Neck	Shoulders

   Breathing   Other:_____

6. What did you do? (Circle the things you did.)

Hit back	Told an adult	Broke something
Ran away	Walked away calmly	Ignored the problem
Yelled	Talked it out	Used Keep Calm
Cried	Talked to my friend	Used Be Your BEST
Cursed	Tried to forget it	Used FIG TESPN

   Other:_____

7. How do you think you handled yourself? (Circle one number.)

1	2	3	4
Great	Pretty good	Okay	Not well at all

8. What would you do next time if it happened again?

---

the last three questions, especially role playing different ways of handling the problem and getting feedback from other members of the group.

The Problem Tracker provides an ideal format for such groups because it helps solve the problem of inconsistent attendance. The format of each group is the same; someone new to the group catches on quite quickly, and students can miss several weeks and still feel comfortable returning to the group because they know what the format will be. Further, by discussing Trackers regularly in groups, students become exposed to a consistent, inductive strategy for thinking through a range of problems and concerns, followed by frequent social skills modeling through the guided rehearsal and practice of alternative actions students might plan to take.

THE STUDENT CONFLICT MANAGER: PROBLEM-SOLVING SOFTWARE FOR DIVERSE APPLICATIONS OF FIG TESPN IN THE COMPUTER AGE

As with most useful innovations, once they are introduced, it appears as if they have been around forever and are indispensable. Such is the case with the application of computer technology to the social decision-making and problem-solving process. At a growing number of schools, one can see students sitting at a computer and addressing not only how to keep out of trouble that they have gotten into, but also how to think through problems they are having with their classes, peers, or health-related or life skills issues.

The Student Conflict Manager/Personal Problem Solving Guide (Psychological Enterprise Incorporated, 1993) is a state-of-the-art, user-friendly technology for helping children resolve problems and make better decisions and choices in all areas of their lives. Today's children have grown up on electronic media. Now, this technology can be used to engage them in improving their own behavior and social skills by learning how to become more effective decision makers and problem solvers.

To get a sense of how computer software can enhance social problem-solving and related social and life skills programs, think about what your school may be missing:

+ A tool for children who are in detention, or other aspects of the discipline system, that, in a constructive way, helps them think through what has gotten them into trouble
+ A way to reach children and help promote thoughtful decision making and problem solving before these kids make irrevocably bad, impulsive, poorly thought-through decisions
+ A way to individualize students' programs more
+ A way to generate more dialoging for individual children than is possible in a large class structure
+ A way to document the problem-solving work that is done with individual students

- Personnel who are available to spend time with children on a regular basis for crisis intervention and prevention
- A tool for training classroom aides, peer counselors, and others new to the social problem-solving approach.

This gives a sense of how this software can be applied.

An Overview of the Student Conflict Manager Software

The Student Conflict Manager/Personal Problem Solving Guide is for professionals who work with children. It provides a technology for guiding students in problem solving and decision making, for both everyday matters and for serious or crisis situations. The Student Conflict Manager/Personal Problem Solving Guide is designed for upper elementary, middle school, and high school students who are facing academic, peer, health-related, teacher, or family problems. It can be used effectively with individuals and in groups.

The Student Conflict Manager/Personal Problem Solving Guide brings ideas, events, feelings, and possibilities into new relationships. It does so by taking the social problem-solving process of dialoging, or facilitative, open-ended questioning, and presenting this to children via the computer. It is based on the set of social problem-solving steps discussed throughout this book. Consistent with the facilitative approach emphasized in earlier chapters, the software program utilizes responses generated and entered by students, rather than a preset list of problems, goals, solutions, and consequences. Extensive prompting by the computer, as well as a focus on the problem from different perspectives, engages even those students who tend to be resistant or minimally expressive.

The set-up for using the Student Conflict Manager/Personal Problem Solving Guide requires an IBM-compatible computer, a 5.25- or 3.5-inch diskette drive, and a printer. The program also can be used on Macintosh computers by combining it with an IBM-based emulator program, such as SoftPC. For ease and independence of use, the computer program has been designed with a minimal number of necessary commands to be performed. These are displayed clearly on the screen; further, context sensitive help is built into the program and is always available by using the Function keys on the keyboard.

Stage I of the program begins with a student typing his or her name and grade level for identification when the work session is printed out. During Stage II, students are asked to identify what happened to get them in trouble or what problem they are thinking about, and they are instructed to be as specific as possible when typing in their responses. Stage II presents a context for the decision making and problem solving to commence and sensitizes the students to look for signs of different feelings, an important skill in the decision-making process.

Stage III is designed to help students consider the problem in a few different ways, and allows them to begin to think of some things they could do about it. For this stage in the process, the computer program has been designed with an algorithm that retrieves text that has already been typed into the program by the student into a new prompt that moves the problem-solving process ahead. For example, students are now asked to list every way they can think of to accomplish the goals that they mentioned during Stage II of the process. The software automatically displays each goal students typed into the program during Stage II and allows them to respond to it. In this way, students begin to develop a list of possible alternative behaviors to the one that got them in trouble. Additionally, the program has been developed to bring up students' responses during Stage II and prompt them to formulate what they can do to keep the behavior from happening again.

During Stage IV, students are able to select from the screen a list of alternative actions that they generated during the computer session. The software automatically compiles the list in a way that can be easily reviewed and prioritized. Figure 6.1 is an example of the computer screen and displays one of the alternative behaviors that has been marked by a student as one of the most realistic strategies to help reach a goal. In the final stage, students are guided through a detailed look at their choices and are given the chance to do some planning about what it will take for their ideas to be carried out realistically and in the face of possible obstacles, or roadblocks.

NEXT STEP	ACTIONS BEING SELECTED
Take a good look at ALL your ideas at the right. Select the ONE that you feel is the BEST. Then select another good one, and another. Only choose a few that you REALLY WANT TO TRY.	1. I could have gotten involved in the discussion I could have apologized ♦Talk about this problem Stay awake

FIGURE 6.1. Simulated personal problem-solving guide screen showing action selected (♦) among alternatives generated.

Preventive Interventions to Help with Everyday Problem Solving, Decision Making, and Conflict Resolution

From a preventive perspective, interventions that would give students a chance to address situations before they faced them would be beneficial. Therefore, one application of the Guide is for students who anticipate a problem and would like to use the computer as an aid to thinking through possible solutions, consequences, and plans. For the clinician, guidance counselor, health educator, school psychologist, social worker, and others engaged in anticipatory guidance and preventive problem solving with children and adolescents, the Guide provides an effective vehicle to structure a problem-solving process, especially for those students who might be reluctant to engage in a direct one-to-one counseling session. It is a useful adjunct to drug and alcohol education programs, to help children think through hypothetical problem situations they might face, to think through how to handle conflicts and resolve disputes, and to rethink situations that they already have faced. In these preventive applications, students need to know about availability of the Guide and to learn how to access it. Some will require an adult to be available to assist them, but many will, after a few sessions, be fully capable of using it largely on their own, as empowered problem solvers.

Addressing Students' Academic Difficulties

Many students experience a common set of problems around organizing themselves to do their academic work. This has been found to be a particular issue around the transition of students into middle, junior high, or high school (Elias, Gara, & Ubriaco, 1985). Another valuable use of the Student Conflict Manager allows teachers, counselors, and learning specialists to help individual students gradually learn to identify aspects of academic organization and related problems and move toward solutions. Several principles underlie the effective use of the program in the context of academic difficulties:

1. Start simple to achieve initial success.
2. Old habits take time to modify and replace with positive work habits.
3. Communication of the Action Plans derived from the program to other educators and to parents can improve consistency and reduce students' frustration.
4. It is important not to stop using the Student Conflict Manager Problem program too soon. Many students still need the "prompt

and cue" value of the software to continue to be successful. Internalization and transfer of learning takes considerable time.

Use of the Student Conflict Manager as Part of Intervention in the Discipline System

Another recent context in which the Student Conflict Manager/Personal Problem Solving Guide has proven valuable is in school discipline systems. When schools adopt the software into their standard practice, students involved in disciplinary infractions can find new ways to resolve their problems. In practice, the student who continually presents to the guidance counselor, school disciplinarian, or principal would work with the Student Conflict Manager/Personal Problem Solving Guide before a discussion would occur. This is likely to take 15 to 20 minutes. The initial times younger students use the Guide, they are likely to need a teacher, aide, or counselor to help keep them on task and to be sure they follow the prompts that are on the screen. Upon completion of the Student Conflict Manager/Personal Problem Solving Guide program, the student would have clarified the problem situation and would have created an alternative set of behaviors, to be used if the student faces a similar situation in the future. More importantly, students who use the Student Conflict Manager/Personal Problem Solving Guide have had the opportunity to be involved in a *constructive* disciplinary activity, which may prevent them from getting into similar difficulties when the same sets of circumstances present themselves.

For many students, the prospect of talking to an adult about their discipline problems is threatening, stressful, anger provoking, or even shameful. The Student Conflict Manager/Personal Problem Solving Guide serves as a welcome "buffer" to a direct confrontation between the student and an adult. It allows a constructive, self-directed review process to begin that leads a student to take greater ownership of the problem and its resolution than usually takes place in a charged disciplinary environment. Similarly, the Guide is a far better use of time in detention or in-school suspension than merely sitting silently or doing seat work.

Research has shown that students using even early versions of the Student Conflict Manager/Personal Problem Solving Guide in detention in middle school were less likely to return to detention because they had a constructive strategy and plan to help cope with the situations that got them into trouble in the first place (Elias & Clabby, 1992). Lickona (1991) also finds that individual conferences leading to an Action Plan are among the most effective techniques for working with hostile students. When one combines the process of inquiry, which conveys respect for students, with the positive time and concern of individual conferencing, Lickona finds that this creates a caring that can be a direct antidote to the disengagement some students strongly feel.

Adults' Roles in Helping Students Turn Their Action Plans into Success

One critical role, of course, is to facilitate students' access to the program, to get them started, and to help them obtain a diskette that will serve as their own personal problem-solving "record." Beyond that, however, adults have an important role in translating ideas into behavior, as would be expected in this variation of a TVDRP approach. The Student Conflict Manager/Personal Problem Solving Guide generates two types of printouts: an Action Plan and a Context Outline. Each has its own use. The Action Plan gives students a list of things that they can do to solve the problem or prevent trouble in the future. The list is based on the ideas that students generated with the Student Conflict Manager/Personal Problem Solving Guide. Because it contains the students' own ideas, the Plan serves as a tangible reminder of behaviors the child is likely to carry out. In addition, some students will have Action Plans that are more detailed and complex, generated by using the part of the program that helps them anticipate and address obstacles to some of their basic plans. The Context Outline is a detailed, printed analysis of the session, including all problem-solving prompts given by the computer and students' responses to them. This can be valuable as a full record of the meeting with the student, which can be entered into relevant school or clinical records or files; it also has been useful for staff members and parents as part of a conference on a particular child.

To increase the likelihood of successful behavioral follow-through, adults can review the Plan prior to the student implementing it. Some students may be unrealistic about what they will be able to do and would therefore benefit from thinking through the plan a little more. The adult may also wish to point out a few obstacles unanticipated by the student, or suggest that the student go on to the obstacles part of the program if he or she has not yet done so. The purpose here is not for the adult to take over the problem-solving process, but to further facilitate students' thinking and planning. Certainly, some students will need to learn first from recognizing ineffective problem solving, and then engaging in the process again (Friedlander, 1993).

Making Students' Plans Realistic

Once the plan is finalized, adults can deepen the process by asking, "Who, what, when, where, and how?" This has been called the politics of problem solving (Clabby & Elias, 1986), and consists of the following types of questions:

- "Who will do this?" "Who else needs to be involved?"
- "What will you do?" "What will you say?" "What else could you say?" "What do you think he will say?"
- "When are you going to do this?" "When are you going to do the next step?" "When are you going to do the other things?"
- "Where will you do this?" "Where else could you do this?"

The "how" can be assisted through guided practice or, in dyadic or group contexts, role playing. As mentioned previously, the more concrete and realistic the experience is for students, the better able they will be to implement their plans in the real world. Have students act out exactly how they would implement their plans, including what they would say, how they would say it, and so forth. The adult can play the other role(s) and re-act as a person might realistically react. Through role plays, certain skill deficits may be noted by the adult, which can be worked on; for example, if a student is going to talk to another student and you notice a need for improvement in eye contact, assertive posture, or tone of voice, it may be necessary to help or arrange for the student to work on these skills prior to an attempt to implement the plan. As mentioned earlier, materials based on the same framework as the Guide are available for this purpose (Elias, 1993; Elias & Clabby, 1989).

In addition, the Action Plan serves as an informal contract. The con-tract can be between the adult and student or even a contract with the stu-dent and him- or herself. Inherent in a contract is the sense of social oblig-ation, as well as a means of monitoring that the obligation has been met. Wherever possible, it is important that someone follow up on the Action Plan to see if and how it was implemented, what the results were, and what further problem solving and planning might be needed. When stu-dents are unable to complete a session, it can be saved to disk and worked on at another time. It is even possible for disks to be taken home by the student to continue the problem-solving process.

Use of the Student Conflict Manager in Counseling and Clinical Situations: A Case Illustration

Tom is a seventh grade student who has been diagnosed as having atten-tion-deficit/hyperactivity disorder (ADHD). He has had both social and academic difficulties in the past. He was referred to the school psycholo-gist after incidents of making obscene comments to several female stu-dents, and one in particular, after being teased by them. The principal who referred Tom was particularly concerned: Tom previously had made other comments that were too loud, disruptive, or annoying to other students, although not to this degree, and Tom did not seem to understand why these comments were not an appropriate response to being teased, despite receiving a 3-day suspension.

Tom met with the school psychologist and discussed his reentry meeting with the principal and his parents. After patient probing and prompting by the psychologist, Tom could verbalize that what he did, as he put it, "crossed the line"; however, due to his impulsive nature, he did not have alternatives for dealing with the girls' teasing. His one solution to the problem was to "ignore them." This was obviously a simplistic solution, probably suggested by his parents. The school psychologist decided to use the Student Conflict Manager to reach Tom in a nonconfrontive, engaging manner. As Tom worked on the Student Conflict Manager, he was encouraged to come up with additional alternatives. This initially took some time, as Tom characteristically wished to impulsively run through the program with few responses. The school psychologist stopped him from advancing to the next screen so quickly, and engaged him to think a little more about it. At times, the school psychologist engaged Tom in a general discussion about the topic on the screen or self-disclosed how he might react to such a situation in order to stimulate Tom's thinking. (Interestingly, Tom was not resistant to stopping and taking more time; it has been found by Student Conflict Manager/Personal Problem Solving Guide users that special needs students often are willing to interface longer and more often with a computer than with a person.) As Tom came up with more responses, he began to understand that there are other ways of seeing and coping with his problem.

Further dialoging around the responses to the Student Conflict Manager led to discussion of nonverbal communication, or "body language." This helped Tom to become aware of more subtle aspects of social communication, and of how this could impact on what he was doing and whether he was going to be successful or not. Other discussions generated during the initial Student Conflict Manager session concerned the girls' motivation for teasing Tom and how one chooses one's friends. (These issues were addressed at a later time using the Problem version of the Student Conflict Manager/Personal Problem Solving Guide.)

In Tom's initial Action Plan, there were numerous spelling and grammatical errors. Because it is important not to take a critical or authoritarian approach when working with the Student Conflict Manager, these errors were not mentioned by the school psychologist as Tom typed them in. In addition, potentially unrealistic options were not endorsed or censored. Tom indicated that one of the things he could have done was to say something "that was a little bit before the line" he had been crossing. Knowing where the line is between appropriate and inappropriate verbalization was Tom's primary interpersonal problem. The school psychologist was aware that Tom did not yet possess the skills needed to make this subtle differentiation. However, this issue was not addressed at this time; to do so would have impeded the process of problem solving. The school psychologist made a note (the Student Conflict Manager/Personal Problem Solving Guide has a Notepad feature to allow this to be incorporated into the program in a background file) to work on this skill, should Tom select it for his Action Plan.

In the second session with the Student Conflict Manager, Tom added in details to the Action Plan in terms of obstacles and how he was going to handle them. The Plan is presented in Table 6.3, uncorrected for typing or grammatical errors. Initially, Tom did not anticipate any obstacles to his "ignoring." This was a key moment for the school psychologist, as a facilitator of students' problem solving, to suggest some possible reactions

TABLE 6.3. Sample Computer-Generated Action Plan with Child's Original Spelling

The Student Conflict Manager/Personal Problem Solving Guide:

TROUBLE

THIS WORKSHEET BELONGS TO:

♦ Tom
♦ Grade 7

WHAT WAS THE TROUBLE?
i got suspended for crossing the line verbly

WHAT I AM GOING TO DO:

Chosen Actions	Handling Obstacles
1. ignore her	♦ she scratches me; i would tell a teacher
	♦ she curses; pretend not to hear her
	♦ I get steaming mad; i would walk away and cool off
2. i could be boringly nice	♦ she thinks I like her; i would tell her that i was going to make plans with people she did not like
	♦ I don't feel like being boringly nice; ignore her
3. i could use body language to let her know i don't want to be her friend	♦ she doesn't see the body language; start talking to my friend and walk away from her

(These are your selected actions with the detailed thinking you have added.)

that the girl might have to being ignored. It was difficult for Tom, as for many children with ADHD, to take the perspective of others and anticipate their reactions. Here, the school psychologist reflected on "human behavior" and gave specific reactions that the girl in question, as well as girls of her age in general, might have. Then, Tom was asked to respond to how he would handle these behaviors, should they take place in response to his actions. This process moves students toward constructive action and helps to inoculate them against failure of their plans by building a sense of realistic expectations. For Tom, prior to anticipating obstacles, he felt either that his actions would always be successful or that he would not be able to handle unexpected reactions. Now, he was being prepared for the girls reaction to him, whatever it might be. (These patterns are familiar to anyone working with special needs students; the problem-solving process anticipates these patterns in a nonconfrontive way.)

The school psychologist and Tom then role played the Action Plan scenarios in order both to assess Tom's ability to implement his ideas and to give him practice doing so. Brief assertiveness training was done as an adjunct to the role playing, using the Be Your BEST technique presented earlier.

After completion of the Student Conflict Manager, and with Tom's permission, the Action Plan (and detailed Context Outline) were shared with the principal. The documentation reassured the principal that Tom was aware of the problem and was working seriously to solve it. Indeed, this record was far more tangible and persuasive than typical reports of having a "good" or "productive" session. The principal noted as well that Tom displayed a greater depth of understanding in the worksheet than had been shown during the principal's discussion with him. The principal then determined that no additional punishments were necessary to help Tom understand the seriousness of his inappropriate behavior. Subsequent sessions between the school psychologist and Tom involved further discussion around this problem, reviews and updates of his Action Plan, addressing additional obstacles, supplementary assertiveness training, and social reinforcement for appropriate problem solving and maintenance of appropriate behavior. There was no recurrence of this or any other behavior problem for Tom for the remainder of the school year.

Additional Uses of the Student Conflict Manager

An instructional dilemma posed for those working with special needs youth is how to balance the necessity for tailored and often individualized practice opportunities with the time demands and the lack of available personnel in the school to provide these opportunities. This is a "person-power" problem all too familiar to those who work with regular or special education services in the schools. Technology often has been alluded to as an aid in solving these kinds of problems, particularly in the future (Jordan, 1993). The Student Conflict Manager was developed specifically to provide a match between a powerful, proven program/instructional approach and computer technology. The software program allows expert assistance to be available to those who want to help students cope with discipline situations and current, anticipated, and even past conflicts, and to come up with alternatives to violence (Elias, Tobias, & Friedlander, 1994).

To carry out such approaches most effectively, it can be helpful to think about a discipline system as a way to get students who have traveled off the main road back onto the highway as quickly as possible. A discipline system should be guided by a principle of "least punitive, most corrective and educational environment possible." Discipline systems also have a triage function; that is, when children are having difficulty with behavior in school, there should a differentiated system to guide them to appropriate services.

In this way, the discipline system does not focus on the population of students who get into detention frequently, whether for violent, aggressive, acting-out behavior or for academic disorganization. Rather, the discipline system takes a school-wide, preventive approach based on an early intervention perspective. The preventive aim is to reduce lost instructional time, prevent dropout, and to promote thoughtful decision making and problem solving before these kids make irrevocably bad, impulsive, poorly thought-through decisions. The early intervention aspect involves school practitioners being alert to early signs of trouble and moving to provide services. The Student Conflict Manager can be the basis of a "family" of early intervention approaches, ranging from serving as an individual "tutorial" for students who need extra practice in problem solving to providing a basis for training peer mediation and conflict resolution providers. Its format is ideal for such purposes, in that diskettes can be taken home and worked on, and brought back in to see what progress was made and, if needed, to print out the Action Plan. A description of some of these uses follows.

Peer Mediation and Conflict Resolution

Training of peer mentors, peer leaders, and conflict managers is a role that school practitioners find themselves taking on (or being given) with increasing frequency (Hechinger, 1992; D. Johnson, Johnson, Dudley, & Burnett, 1992; Willis, 1993) With the Student Conflict Manager, a trainer can give potential mentors and peer leaders standardized or tailored problems and examine the nature of their problem-solving process. Patience and persistence, as well as skill levels, can be seen clearly. Such training also can go on in a group format, with the use of an LCD overhead projector to which a computer is connected or by using the video output capacity of many computers and projecting a problem or conflict onto a large television monitor so that groups of students can see it more easily than they can see a computer screen.

The Prereferral Social Problem Solving Lab

The Social Problem Solving (SPS) Lab is a prereferral intervention format that has been quite successful in its initial applications (Nigro, 1995). The Lab consists of a room in which one finds a computer, a school practitioner acting as a facilitator (and/or supervising a trained Intern, student teacher, or paraprofessional who acts in that role), and the Student Conflict Manager diskettes for individual students. As it has been used in pilot tests, the procedure involves teachers, guidance counselors, and other pupil services personnel deciding on some criteria that will indicate that a student is having persistent behavioral, learning-related, or self-organizational problems that, if they were to persist, might warrant a referral for special education classification. When such behavior is seen, the child is referred at this relatively early stage to the SPS Lab. There, the child is encouraged to work with the Student Conflict Manager to explore the problem. The computer would be there, as would posters made by children depicting the social problem-solving steps and other important related skills such as Keep Calm and Be Your BEST. Over several sessions, these individuals work with children on problems identified by the classroom teachers, other school personnel, or even the children themselves. The children would be shown how to "dialog" with the computer.

An important feature of the Lab is that the software can produce an Action Plan. Having something tangible, in one's hands, that represents one's own work is highly reinforcing for students. The written plan also is a valuable tool for documenting the work done in counseling—that is, the SPS Lab—and provides a clear way to share with school staff and parents just what it is that the child is working on. Thus, the key adults in the child's life can be a team of problem-solving facilitators. (Particularly for high school students, there is an advanced subroutine of the program that allows children to anticipate obstacles to their Action Plan and generate a more detailed written plan that includes how they would handle any roadblocks that might come up.)

When the process moves into the planning and enactment stage, the staff member in the Lab will do rehearsal and practice with the student. This itself often is diagnostic, as children display combinations of anxiety or interpersonal skill problems that indicate some on-the-spot instruction in Keep Calm or BEST might be appropriate. Also, when several children are at the same stage, that is, they have developed Action Plans and have practiced with staff, it is valuable to have them work in pairs or small groups, share their solutions and plans, practice with one another, and give and get feedback in one more "dress rehearsal" performance before trying their solutions with the real audience in place. Consistent with the FIG TESPN model, follow-up sessions to discuss the "next time" and how the plans or their implementation might need changing, or just to validate their effectiveness and be sure kids give themselves the proper credit for their problem-solving expertise, are scheduled routinely. The SPS Lab has been used with students as young as third graders; with older students, especially in high school, it also is valuable to have ways they can access the program and computers on their own, such as during a free period or study hall. However, some students have been helped by having "passes" that allow them to leave a class and go and use the Student Conflict Manager when they find they are particularly upset or feel as if they might lose self-control.

In a recent pilot test in a racially diverse school for grades 3–5 in the Northeast, administrative records showed that children who were referred to the SPS Lab were those who otherwise would have been discussed for referral to child study team evaluation. The administrators concluded that the SPS Lab was effective as a "prereferral intervention." Data gathered by Nigro (1995) showed that students in the Lab made considerable skills gains, thus reinforcing the observations of the administrators.

General Evidence for Effectiveness

The Student Conflict Manager/Personal Problem Solving Guide operationalizes the social decision-making and problem-solving process presented earlier. Over a decade of research has shown that interventions using this approach with diverse student populations, including special needs students in schools and residential treatment centers, have improved students' peer relationships, self-esteem, and ability to cope with stressors. In the long-term, it reduces students' risk of involvement with alcohol, delinquency, and related problem behaviors (Elias, 1983; Elias, Gara, Schuyler, Branden-Muller, & Sayette, 1991). Most specifically, in addition to case study examples, It should be noted that the specific social decision-making and problem-solving steps used as the basis of the Guide were developed over a number of years, combining clinical and school observations of aspects of interpersonal decision making and problem solving that, when deficient, were associated with problem behaviors and other indices of poor adjustment. The steps' application in a variety of contexts is well documented, through both clinical treatment and curriculum-based modalities (Elias & Clabby, 1992). The Student Conflict Manager/Personal Problem Solving Guide appears to provide a constructive approach to intervention that builds students' skills and increases the likelihood of generalization to everyday behaviors and situations. Further, the program provides the structure and feedback that gives special needs students a much-cherished bolstering of their sense of self-efficacy and of the belief that they are capable of problem solving effectively for themselves. Work is currently being completed on developing the Parenting and Family Problem Solving Guide, a version of the software that will allow parents to use the social problem-solving approaches in their households with all family members about school and other issues, as well as to sort out the way parents are coping with their various parenting problems and dilemmas.

CHAPTER 7

♦♦♦

Incorporating Social Problem Solving within School Routines and Mandates

♦

At the heart of life skills teaching, for all youngsters, disadvantaged and advantaged alike, must be the recognition that they stand at the threshold of greater independence and responsibility for their futures [i.e., they stand poised ready to become responsible citizens and contributing members of workplaces, institutions of learning, community and families]. The decisions they will soon have to make have lifelong consequences for themselves and others; decisions about their education and goals, about smoking, drinking, and drugs, about the use of vehicles, and, tragically, even decisions about the use of weapons. Knowledge [and skills] for the making of judgments can be taught. It is a great mistake to assume that young people will acquire these skills automatically.

—*Hechinger (1992, p. 128)*

This chapter addresses ways in which school practitioners can bring social problem-solving strategies into students' everyday school routines and mandated activities. Specifically, approaches will be provided that can be infused (1) into language arts and literature; (2) as a part of social studies, history, and current events instruction; (3) during health and family life education, especially substance abuse prevention; and (4) when projects or reports are required in any subject area. Particular attention is given to examples that embrace the increasing emphasis on multicultural education and acceptance of diversity, and the growing reality of inclusive education in our classrooms and schools.

These applications gain their potency through repetition and coordination. Activities that may be interesting to students but lack a common thread are given that cognitive connection by having the steps of FIG TESPN embedded within them. The clearest example of this is current events, where the use of social problem-solving infusion, as described below, not only helps students become more familiar with the events going on around them, but also gives them a strategy to use when they encounter local, national, and international events personally or through the media.

Coordination refers to the benefits of students' having converging cognitive approaches in different academic areas, such as health and language arts. This becomes especially important to children from diverse cultures, in that it allows them to pick up on a consistent framework for learning and thinking, and to children with special education classifications, in that it reduces the amount of cognitive integration and differentiation they have to do as they try to sort out the various implicit instructional paradigms they encounter in various classes and subject areas.

LANGUAGE ARTS AND LITERATURE

When reading a story, students can apply the FIG TESPN framework to problems that are encountered or decisions that the characters make (Naftel & Elias, 1995). In doing this, it is important to start with a discussion of how the characters feel about a certain situation. This requires a high degree of inferential thinking at times. Students can then identify the problem and goal in their own words, which also facilitates reading comprehension. Students can see that there may be other options that can be taken by the characters in the story. These options and potential outcomes can be discussed. If the character had a plan, this too can be evaluated by the students. Finally, it may be interesting for students to infer what happens after the story ends. These topics can either be discussed in class or done as written assignments. Table 7.1 lists a secondary-level and a beginning set of "Book Talk" guidelines for bringing these ideas into language arts and literature classes.

School practitioners can take advantage of formats like this by assisting teachers to carry out these procedures as a regular part of their language arts program. However, the creation of such things as Book Talk clubs, literary review magazines and clubs, and the like provide school practitioners with innovative and stigma-free ways to build academic, interpersonal, and social problem-solving skills with at-risk youth. Other types of assignments or discussions involve having students read or hear part of a story and then using FIG TESPN to complete it, giving students

TABLE 7.1. Questions Assigned to Students in Problem Solving Applied to Literature Analysis/Book Talks

1. Think of an event in the section of the book assigned. When and where did it happen? Put the event into words as a problem.

2. Who were the people that were involved in the problem? What were their different feelings and points of view about the problem? Why did they feel as they did? Try to put their goals into words.

3. For each person or group of people, what are some different decisions or solutions to the problem that he, she, or they thought of that might help in reaching their goals?

4. For each of these ideas or options, what are all of the things that might happen next? Envision and write down short- and long-term consequences.

5. What were the final decisions? How were they made? By whom? Why? Do you agree or disagree? Why?

6. How was the solution carried out? What was the plan? What obstacles were met? How well was the problem solved? What did you read that supports your point of view?

7. Notice what happened and re-think it. What would you have chosen to do? Why?

8. What questions do you have, based on what you read? What questions would you like to be able to ask one or more of the characters? The author? Why are these questions important to you?

Simplified Book Talk Format for Young Readers

I will write about this character . . .

My character's problem is . . .

How did your character get into this problem . . .

How does the character feel?

What does the character want to happen?

What questions would you like to be able to ask the character you picked, one of the other characters, or the author?

---

the beginning and end of stories and then requiring them to make up a middle, or using FIG TESPN for increasing the creativity and careful checking that goes into creative writing projects (see Elias & Clabby, 1989).

Issues of authors' styles, paraphrasing, and use of language can be highlighted with adolescents and preadolescent gifted and talented students. An analysis can be made of the authors' purposes in having plans crafted as they did, and meeting the outcomes they did. Issues of dramatic tension, irony, and conflict all can be illustrated easily. Finally, it may be interesting for students to infer what happens after a story ends. Perhaps sequels can be discussed, outlined, or written.

SOCIAL STUDIES INSTRUCTION

The Perspective of Persons and Groups Engaging in Historically Based Decisions

Among many perspectives for social studies (or social sciences) instruction, one that we have found highly engaging to students emphasizes how decisions have been, and continue to be, made in the context of history. Both history and current events can be thought of as a series of decisions made by individuals and groups, often in response to actual or anticipated problems, reflecting certain goals, options, consequences, plans, and lessons for the future. Table 7.2 applies this idea and shows an adaptation of FIG TESPN for use in current events instruction. Consider how often current events are discussed in the schools without any systematic framework to provide a unifying cognitive frame to use outside these school-based discussions. Current events lessons are an opportune time for school practitioners to work with students and also introduce teachers to the academic benefits of FIG TESPN and social problem solving.

An example of a FIG TESPN used as a framework for analyzing historical events can be found in Table 7.3. This application, as well as a variation used in the creation of a newspaper club for students, has been

---

TABLE 7.2. Thinking about Current Events

1. What is the event that you are thinking about? When and where is it happening? Put the event into words as a problem, choice, or decision.

2. What people or groups were involved in the problem? What are their different feelings? What are their points of view about the problem?

3. What do each of these people or groups want to have happen? Try to put their goals into words.

4. For each person or group, name some different options or solutions to the problem that they think might help them reach their goals. Add any ideas that you think might help them that they might not have thought of.

5. For each option or solution you listed, picture all the things that might happen next. Envision long- and short-term consequences.

6. What do you think the final decision should be? How should it be made? By whom? Why?

7. Imagine a plan to help you carry out your solution. What could you do or think of to make your solution work? What obstacles or roadblocks might keep your solution from working? Who might disagree with your ideas? Why? What else could you do?

8. Rethink it. Is there another way of looking at the problem that might be better? Are there other groups, goals, or plans that come to mind?

TABLE 7.3. Thinking about Important Events in History

1. What is the event that you are thinking about? When and where did it happen? Put the event into words as a problem, choice, or decision.

2. What people or groups were involved in the problem? What were their different feelings? What were their points of view about the problem?

3. What did each of these people or groups want to have happen? Try to put their goals into words.

4. For each person or group, name some different options or solutions to the problem that they thought might help them reach their goals.

5. For each option or solution, picture all the things that might have happened next. Envision both long- and short-term consequences.

6. What were the final decisions? How were they made? By whom? Why? Do you agree or disagree? Why?

7. How was the solution carried out? What was the plan? What obstacles or road-blocks were met? How well was the problem solved? Why?

8. Rethink it. What would you have chosen to do? Why?

shown to improve students' social studies skills (Haboush & Elias, 1993). Other successfully used social studies outlines based on FIG TESPN can be found in Elias and Clabby (1989). All of these outlines also link well with readings, further research, and various types of projects.

Civics, Citizenship, and Education for Democracy

This perspective is compatible with recent compilations of resources in the area of civics and citizenship education, such as *CIVITAS* (Quigley & Bahmueller, 1991) and *Civics for Democracy* (Isaac, 1992). The former provides K–12 scope and sequence and detailed content outlines in areas such as civic virtue, civic participation, the nature of politics and government in the United States, the role of the citizen, and fundamental values and principles of the United States. Throughout all of these areas, a strong historical perspective is taken, and applications to present issues are obvious. Such applications are readily apparent in Isaac's (1992) format, as she focuses on citizen movements such as civil rights, labor, women's rights, and environmentalism. Focused at the high school level, *Civics for Democracy* includes many case studies and activity and worksheet ideas. Schools run by religious organizations also tend to focus on civics as taught from their particular value system; the worksheets in Tables 7.2 and 7.3 and Probe (Table 4.2) can be applied in religious education contexts as well (e.g., Gopin, Levine, & Schwartz, 1994).

Incorporating Historically Based Readings

Social problem-solving frameworks articulate well with social studies literature at all grade levels (Alexander & Crabtree, 1988). For young readers, books such as *Watch the Stars Come Out* by Riki Levinson (in the Reading Rainbow Library edition, published by E.P. Dutton) contain stories that relate to historical periods (here, the immigration from Europe to the "Land of Liberty") and complementary enrichment activities. Older readers may enjoy anthologies that focus not only on history but America's diversity, such as, *In the Spirit of Peace* (Defense for Children–International, New York), *Goodbye Vietnam* (Alfred A. Knopf, New York), *Growing Up Asian American* (William Morrow & Co., New York), and *Visions of America: Personal Narratives from the Promised Land* (Persea Books, New York). A continuing source of information in this area is the magazine *Teaching Tolerance*, published by the Southern Poverty Law Center.

At many points, FIG TESPN can be used to help students think more deeply about the issues presented in these and other sources (e.g., How did immigrants feel about leaving their countries? What countries were they leaving? What problems were going on that made them want to leave? What problems would leaving bring about? What would have been their goals in leaving or staying? What were their options and how did they envision the results of each possibility? What plans did they have to make? What kinds of things got in their way at the last minute? How did they overcome the roadblocks? Once they arrived how did they feel? What problems did they encounter at the beginning? What were their first goals? etc.). As needed, further reading and research could be assigned to help students find fact-based answers to these and related questions, in addition to checking their own thoughts.

A powerful unit can be done for children with regard to readings concerning historical and cultural events, such as the Holocaust. The use of facilitative questioning can help students focus on the feelings expressed by the writers, understand the writers' points of view, understand the frame of reference of the characters in the texts, and create a work of their own, in the form of a fictionalized story or poem, that captures their feelings, thoughts, and questions about these horrific events. Recent books that can serve as the anchors for such a unit include the following:

+ Susan Bachrach, *Tell Them We Remember* (Little, Brown, New York) [combines history and personal stories to teach young readers through the tragic accounts of 20 children and their families who survived the Holocaust]
+ Children of Terezin, *I Never Saw Another Butterfly* (Schocken, New York) [a collection of poems and drawings of children from the Terezin concentration camp]

◆ Carol Matas, *Daniel's Story* (Scholastic, New York) [based on a permanent exhibition at the United States Holocaust Memorial Museum in Washington, DC, it tells a fictional account of a courageous young boy and his family and their struggle to survive]

Creating Student Action Groups

Beginning around middle school age, an exciting offshoot of the social problem-solving and decision-making approach is to have teams of students organize using FIG TESPN as a framework to address and resolve genuine problems. These could be problems in the school, local community issues, or even larger problems of pollution, war and peace, world hunger, and lack of liberty. In the Berkeley Heights, New Jersey, school district, sixth grade students addressed local environmental problems using the approaches suggested here. The students' received community-wide attention, recognition by the state legislature, and the project culminated in a Presidential Environmental Award, complete with a White House ceremony (Johnson & Bruene-Butler, 1993).

The idea of organizing students as problem-solving teams using FIG TESPN fits with and is complementary to many recent curricular initiatives related to the "global community" and such topics as vandalism, poverty, education, world peace, terrorism, toxic wastes, future jobs, and the elderly (Crabbe, 1989; DeBock & Paul, 1989; Kniep, 1986). For high school students, a challenging application of this work is to participate in the nonpartisan Foreign Policy Association's *Great Decisions* series (729 Seventh Avenue, New York, NY 10019). Each year, a briefing book, activities book, bibliography, leadership handbook, and world map are developed around key topics. The materials are designed to provide information for discussion and to assist in developing school-wide and community forums and communication with policy makers.

APPLICATIONS TO HEALTH AND FAMILY LIFE EDUCATION

Health educators, to an increasing degree, are identifying sound decision making around health-related behaviors as an overarching instructional goal (Irwin, 1987; Kolbe, 1985; Purdy & Tritsch, 1985). Social decision making—including skills related to self-control, social awareness, and group participation—is well suited to serve as a basic, integrative, developmental framework for health-related decision making. It is most useful when "health" is defined to include physical, social, community, familial, or psychological aspects, as is recommended by the National Professional

School Health Organizations (1984; Jessor, 1991). Although there are many effective ways to accomplish an infusion of social problem solving and decision making into health education, we will focus on these following: (1) FIG TESPN as a guide for health-related discussions, (2) a TV-DRP format for covering health topics, and (3) a language arts format for generating critical thinking and discussion around health issues.

FIG TESPN: Tackling the Problem of Alcohol, Tobacco, and Other Drug Use

Use and abuse of alcohol, tobacco, steroids, and other drugs, like all health-related issues, must be labeled for students as reflecting both personal and interpersonal decisions. Every health behavior has effects on oneself and on others (friends, classmates, parents, siblings, other relatives) and the effects must be carefully separated, specified, and examined. Any given substance—cigarettes, chewing tobacco, beer, wine, hard liquor, pills, steroids, cocaine, crack, heroin, amphetamines, barbiturates, and so forth—can be introduced and discussed using FIG TESPN as a framework. One way to open such a discussion is, "How do you feel when (or, would you feel if) someone asks you to try _____ ?" Different ways of thinking through the problem can be put on the board or written down; possible consequences and obstacles of trying different solutions and plans can be tried out through guided practice and rehearsal.

A more general way of introducing such discussions with younger children is to ask, "How do you feel about . . . (e.g., cigarettes)?" "What problems do you see for people who smoke?" Then, goals can be set, alternatives to smoking discussed, and plans made. As part of the last step in FIG TESPN, students can be asked to make public commitments about not smoking, an effective public health technique. Among the youngest students, teachers find it useful to ask them to discuss how FIG TESPN would advise people who are thinking about smoking or alcohol or drugs. How do you think FIG feels about smoking? Why? What does smoking do to your body? What problems would FIG point out? How would FIG want that person's health to turn out? What would FIG suggest someone do instead of smoke? If someone bothered you to smoke, how would FIG want you to handle it? and so on. FIG TESPN also is useful for discussing the related, delicate problem of what to do when a friend or loved one is involved in some form of substance abuse. This is a volatile issue, especially when a parent is involved.

Across all health-related FIG TESPN applications, the most important skills to emphasize are to guide oneself with clear goals and to envision a variety of outcomes, or consequences. Everyone has goals; however, goals often are not articulated and therefore do not serve as clear guides for behavior. In addition, there are long- and short-term goals that may conflict. Therefore, as discussions take place, the following incomplete sentences can be put on the board and used to keep track of goals that students express:

"When people_____, their goal is to_____."

Some examples include, "When people eat vegetables, their goal is to please their parents"; "When people drink beer, their goal is to be part of the group"; "When people spend time with their families, their goal is to have fun being with them."

The link of actions, goals, and consequences can then be made by creating workstations that look something like this:

If my goal is to_____, then some things that can help me get there and not hurt me or others are: _____

_____

_____

_____."

For each goal, a "menu" or personal workbook can be created that students can review and have available to add to or look over for ideas throughout the year. Teachers often find it useful to provide a set of goals that are the common implicit or hidden reasons that contribute to high-risk health behaviors. These include the following:

* to fit into a group
* to please one's friends
* to relieve "pressure"
* to imitate sports stars
* to feel good or happy
* to imitate television, video, or music personalities
* to get revenge on parents (or others)

By placing these goals in the format of the worksheet, the idea of using risky health behaviors to reach these goals loses some of its plausibility and secrecy.

Many schools use existing health promotion or substance abuse prevention curricula or programs. Teachers find that FIG TESPN is highly consistent with virtually all such programs because it provides a consistent framework for thinking and decision making that can be applied across individual topic areas. The resulting curricular continuity and synergy makes it more likely that instructional goals can be met. Examples of health programs and curricula related to substance abuse that articulate well with FIG TESPN include *Growing Healthy* (National Center for Health Education, 1985), Life Skills Training (Botvin, 1985), AIDS prevention (Centers for Disease Control, 1988, as well as those developed by local Departments of Education), the *Nutrition Education Curriculum* (Cornell Cooperative Extension, 1989), the *Minnesota Smoking Prevention Program* (Halper, Klepp, Murray, Perry, & Smyth, 1986), *Programs to Advance Teen Health* (PATH; Oregon Research Institute, 1986), and the *Teenage Health Teaching Modules* (Educational Development Center, 1994). Self-control, social awareness, and group participation skills also are valuable adjuncts to these and related curricula (Elias & Clabby, 1989).

TVDRP: Addressing the Transition to Adolescence

The topic of transition to adolescence encompasses many different aspects of health; the situations faced by students as they negotiate their transitions lead to innumerable decisions and problems. The TVDRP format is an engaging way to organize a series of lessons—in classroom or group contexts—relating to the transition. The video material can come from a variety of sources; many public television stations broadcast excellent series, and companies like the Agency for Instructional Technology (1994) are constantly developing and updating relevant series. Contemporary movies or television shows can be used, if screened carefully beforehand. Either a video that touches upon a variety of problem areas, several that focus on specific topics, or a combination can be used. In each case, the video provides a springboard for focused discussion, rehearsal, practice, and other follow-up activities. Table 7.4 contains an instructional outline, based on a TVDRP approach, to be used to explore the transition to adolescence and to be adapted for other health-related purposes; no single specific video is needed for this activity. Subsequent lessons, some using TVDRP, others using FIG TESPN, and others using the language arts and Taming Tough Topics approaches to be described next, would focus on specific health-related topics generated in the discussion.

Language Arts and Social Problem Solving: Partners in Promoting Health

Children enjoy reading stories, and stories are a valuable way to build language skills, encourage thoughtful social decision making, and apply both sets of skills to health and family life issues. Also, a wider range of students find stories more engaging then they do more didactic and text-based health-related presentations. Stories can be read and discussed from the overall FIG TESPN perspective presented in Table 2.2 or the literature

TABLE 7.4. Outline of TVDRP Introduction to Transition to Adolescence: Becoming an Adolescent—New Feelings, New Decisions

Purpose

1. To help students acknowledge, label, and share the new feelings they are experiencing as they enter into adolescence.
2. To help students acknowledge, label, and share the kinds of problems they are now facing as they enter into adolescence.
3. To help students see that these new feelings and the new problems that arise provide opportunities for making decisions.
4. To introduce the concept of understanding the *goals* they have in a given situation.

Instructional Outline

1. *Prepare*
   a. Elicit some of the changes involved in becoming an adolescent by asking students to share some problems they have had to deal with since they started (fifth, sixth, seventh) grade or to share some changes in their feelings; OR
   b. Assign students to read about some of the changes involved in becoming an adolescent prior to any discussion.
2. *Review*
   a. Ask students to recall any previous class work on this topic.
3. *Orient*
   a. Make the point that handling the feelings, problems, and opportunities that go along with becoming an adolescent involves *making decisions and solving problems.* Ask them what it means to be a *thoughtful decision maker and problem solver* and list these qualities on the board.
   b. Make the point that feelings and problems don't "make" us do things—*we* decide and *we* choose. We can do a better job of choosing if we are thoughtful decision makers. (If students have learned social problem solving and decision making and/or FIG TESPN, review these skills with them and point out their relevance to adolescent decisions.)
   c. Use examples from health and personal care (care of teeth, taking vitamins or medicine, smoking) and ask: "How do you decide whether or not to _____?"
4. *Focus*
   a. Tell the class that today you are going to watch a videotape about _____ (e.g., a segment from programs about children entering into adolescence, such as episodes of the *The Cosby Show, The Wonder Years, DeGrassi Junior High,* or *My So-Called Life*).
   b. Ask half the students to focus on all the different problems the focal character is having and ask the other half to focus on all the feelings the focal character expresses.
5. *Show*
   a. Show the videotape.

(continued)

117

TABLE 7.4 *(continued)*

6. *Discuss*

   a. Review the main events and sequence of the video.

   b. Ask students to report the focal character's problems; ask someone to list them on the board.

   c. Ask students to report the feelings they noticed, and the signs of those feelings; ask someone to list them on the board.

   d. Say that sometimes our feelings and problems make it confusing to figure out what to do. When this happens, we have to think about our goals—what we want to have happen. Ask how the focal character felt during each problem and what his or her *goal* might be; what would *the students'* goals be if *they* were the focal character?

7. *Rehearse and practice*

   a. Set up opportunities to rehearse how they might try to reach different goals if they were the focal character. Give different actors a chance to try each situation. (If students know Be Your BEST or other social skills prompts, encourage their use.)

   b. Offer students the opportunity to talk about, rehearse, and practice problems *they* have been facing. Assist the class in offering constructive feedback.

8. *Summarize*

   Regardless of the stopping point for this activity, elicit summaries of what has been happening and the main points learned; correct as needed. Prepare students for the next meeting.

9. *Continue*

   a. Plan follow-up activities, either focusing on one aspect of adolescent changes or on a range of changes. Encourage small group work and projects.

   b. Provide worksheets with different situations and ask students to list possible feelings and goals for different decisions. Ask students to work individually or in groups, and use decisions like these:

   ◆ What time to go to sleep (early or late)
   ◆ Whether to clean your room (yes or no)
   ◆ Whether to smoke (yes or no)
   ◆ How to handle all your energy (work or play)
   ◆ How to handle it when a boy/girl you like ignores you (sad, angry, persistent)
   ◆ Whether to take something from a store if your friends are also doing it (yes or no)
   ◆ Whether to cheat on a test or copy someone else's work and hand it in (yes or no)
   ◆ Whether to drink alcohol (yes or no)

   The format of the worksheet could ask about feelings and goals for each possible decision (e.g., "What would be your feelings and goals if you said 'Yes, I will keep my room clean?' What would be your feelings and goals if you said, 'No, I won't keep my room clean?'").

   c. Hand out a sheet to help students keep track of feelings, problems, goals, decisions, and reasons for their chosen actions, around problem situations that come up during the next two days. These can be reviewed as part of the *presentation* and *review* sections of the next meeting.

   d. Assign a language arts follow-up activity (described in the text).

analysis format presented in Table 7.1; students can be asked to focus on (1) examining how different characters were feeling, (2) analyzing how the author conveyed those feelings, (3) clarifying characters' goals, (4) exploring various options and consequences (both those presented and those *not* presented), and (5) designing alternative endings. Stories can be read through or discussions can be held at appropriate points, perhaps anticipating certain choices and decisions. Examples of stories and topics for young readers include *Little Rabbit's Loose Tooth* (dental) by Lucy Bate, *Bea and Mr. Jones* (the world of work) by Amy Schwartz, *The Sleep Book* (sleep and rest) by Dr. Seuss, *So That's How I Was Born* (conception and birth) by Dr. Richard Brooks; *Gregory The Terrible Eater* (nutrition) by Mitchell Shermat, and *Arthur's Eyes* (glasses, vision, handicaps) by Marc Brown.

For middle schoolers, useful books include *My Life in the Seventh Grade* (general problems) by Mark Geller, as well as assorted books by Judy Blume, Mary Stolz, Miriam Chaikin, John Fitzgerald, Roald Dahl, and Erich Kastner (each has written about a variety of problem areas and issues). In addition, short articles from various magazines (*Highlights, Cricket, Humpty Dumpty, World*) can be useful springboards for language arts lessons. Appendix A contains an example of how independent story-reading assignments can be crafted to focus on key health-decision making skills, using original, interrelated stories for middle schoolers based on the theme, "Think Now for Later". Each set of stories can lead to writing assignments and/or whole class or small group discussions, based on structured questions or general thought-essays.

For high schoolers, Bill Cosby's books (*Fatherhood, Time Flies, Love and Marriage*) offer insights and humor, and opportunities to check out his views and put forth alternative perspectives about family living, parenting, raising teenagers, and parents' own adult development and aging. Other books include Ryan White's *My Own Story*, about his fight against AIDS; Judy Blume's *Starring Sally J. Friedman as Herself*; T. Johnson's *A Rock and a Hard Place*, also about a teen's fight against AIDS, as well as overcoming an abusive childhood; and R. Peck's *Close Enough to Touch*, about a teenager who has to cope with his girlfriend's death.

A SOCIAL PROBLEM-SOLVING FORMAT FOR PLANNING AND CARRYING OUT PROJECTS AND REPORTS

Among many skills needed for social and academic success, one that is given too little instructional emphasis is the process of planning and carrying out projects and reports. Such a process can invoke rote procedures geared toward "getting finished" or it can be one that engages and promotes critical thinking. Diverse groups of learners, including those with special education classifications, respond well when they have a choice about (1) what it is within a topic they will focus on, (2) where they will look for information, and (3) how they will present it. The worksheet in Table 7.5, Taming Tough Topics, is based on a highly successful lesson plan for accomplishing the above purposes (Elias & Clabby, 1989, pp. 157–158).

Taming Tough Topics recognizes that, although a topic often must be determined by the teacher, at times there can be, and should be, some latitude to explore aspects of that topic. Similarly, too often students are channeled toward a standard written report. This tends to lead to an excursion to an encyclopedia or CD-ROM for some copying. For some students with poor writing skills, written reports can be a guaranteed—and unnecessary—turn-off.

Given some choice, students become more motivated to expend effort. In one special education class using Taming Tough Topics as a framework for studying the topic of Native Americans of New Jersey, students wanted to learn more about what happened to the Indians, the

TABLE 7.5. Taming Tough Topics Outline

First: Define your problem and goal.

1. What is the topic?
2. What are some questions you would like to answer about the topic, or some things about the topic you would like to learn?

Second: List alternative places to look for information.

1. Write at least five possible places where you can look for information.

    a. _____

    b. _____

    c. _____

    d. _____

    e. _____

2. Plan which ones you will try first.
3. If these ideas do not work, who else can you ask for ideas? Where else can you look for information?

Third: List alternative ways to present the topic.

1. Write at least three ways in which to present the topic. If it is a written report, write three different ways it can be put together.
2. Consider the consequences for each way, choose your best solution, and plan how you will do it.

Fourth: Make a final check, and fix what needs fixing.

Does your presentation answer the topic and the questions you asked? Is it clear and neat? Is the spelling correct? Will others enjoy what you have done?

sports they played, even the radio station they listened to. They generated places to look for information that included museums, sound filmstrips, and finding people of Native American ancestry. Their presentation formats ranged from a written interview with an Indian to a series of dioramas to a "period play"; older students also have created videos. Typically, teachers review the Taming Tough Topics worksheet with a group or an entire class, brainstorming answers to each question and writing them on the board. This engages students in a shared social problem-solving process, and this process continues as they select their own preferences and then carefully plan and check their work before deciding their final product is completed.

Applications of Taming Tough Topics

AIDS

One fascinating use of Taming Tough Topics has been around AIDS. As a means of gauging students' knowledge and concerns, educators have introduced the topic of AIDS, and then engaged classes or other groups of students in grades K through 12 in discussions of the various questions. Based on the responses, developmentally and informationally appropriate assignments have been generated, ranging from a simple focus ("What is it?") to the more philosophical ("Why do people have to die from it?") to the extremely difficult ("Why do some people survive it?"). The projects that result, when shared among classmates, capitalize on the benefits of peer mediated learning and evoke visibly engaged, interested responses.

Inclusion

Another use of Taming Tough Topics has been as a vehicle for preparing classes for inclusive education. In one situation, an autistic child was going to join a third-grade class. The class used Taming Tough Topics as a way to learn about autism, and by the time the student was ready to enter the class, the class was ready for him. They not only had an understanding of autism, but also of how best to include the child in the classroom and to respond to him during difficult times. Relatedly, self-contained special education classes and individual students with handicapping conditions have had their perspectives broadened considerably through applications of Taming Tough Topics. Some special education classes actually turn their work into presentations to educate other members of the school community. Taming Tough Topics also can be used to guide consultation with staff members. For example, it is not only students who need to be prepared for inclusion of a special education student; staff members also need information and ways to deal effectively with the child, group dynamics in the class and school, and with parents. The Taming Tough Topics format can be useful for individual or group consultation. (Additional considerations in consultation will be discussed in Chapter 8.)

Violence and Cultural Diversity

An additional area of application of Taming Tough Topics has been difficult school issues. One of particular relevance has been violence in the school. School practitioners can have an especially valuable role here by having students do Taming Tough Topics on the use of guns and other weapons in the schools, especially because such issues often are uncomfortable for school personnel to discuss directly with their students. School-wide discussions, resolutions, and rules can follow from various separate groups carrying out and sharing their Taming Tough Topics work. Other areas in which a similar approach has been beneficial include suicide and attempted suicide; racial, ethnic, and cultural stereotyping and prejudice; and other separating aspects of schools, such as tracking.

Famous People

Relatedly, the importance of role models in students' learning is substantial. This can be capitalized on through the medium of written biographies. Taming Tough Topics can be an excellent vehicle for teaching students about the details—especially the hard work, determination, commitment, and other skills—that are part of the successes of the people they find admirable. Biographical information on figures such as Martin Luther King, Jr.; many of the Presidents; explorers, inventors, and scientists such as Ben Franklin and Marie Curie; entertainment figures such as Walt Disney, Gloria Estefan, Leonard Bernstein, and Judith Jamison bring to life the realities of success, as well as certain historical periods. Along with the work of Taming Tough Topics, when classes or groups are reading the same things, FIG TESPN can be used to discuss the focal individual's feelings, goals, alternatives, and the like at various points in his or her life. Throughout this and other activities in this chapter, the focus is on building students' thinking abilities and social problem-solving and decision-making skills—which are essential for functioning effectively in a sophisticated, 21st-century society.

CHAPTER 8

♦♦♦

Program Adaptation
and Staff Training

♦

As our country's schools incorporate increasingly diverse student
populations, the old definitions of excellence are challenged by
the competing values, styles, and frames of intelligences of people
from different origins.

—*Lawrence (1989, p. 15)*

At least 80% of the students in this country, like every other
country in the world, have never acquired what you and I would
agree is one of the major ingredients of being a well educated
person: the capacity to use their minds well. . . . To engage a
mind in school, to get some students to be passionately engaged in
school, is the heart of a good education.

—*Meier (1989, pp. 25–26)*

Social problem-solving techniques have been applied to a variety of populations, from preschoolers to adults, and for a variety of reasons, such as
developing greater social competence, coping with environmental stress,
and solving interpersonal conflicts. FIG TESPN is a generic format that
can be used across settings; however, those working with specific populations and programs have found it beneficial to make appropriate adaptations and modifications. This chapter discusses some examples of those
adaptations, describes issues in consultation and staff training that one
must take into consideration when introducing and using social problem
solving in different school populations, and concludes with an overview of
ways to involve parents in supporting the social problem-solving work being done in school.

TAILORING SOCIAL PROBLEM SOLVING
TO DIFFERENT POPULATIONS

Learning Disabled Populations

Children with learning disabilities often have deficits in social skills. They have difficulty reading nonverbal and other subtle social cues. They can be rejected by peers, and this can compound their feelings of failure, which are often associated with academic frustration. Social skill development is a crucial area for these children and is often included in the individualized education program. When addressed, social skills are often taught in a resource room or other pullout program; it is also necessary to address social skills in mainstreamed settings and in less structured environments such as the lunchroom and the playground.

When working with learning disabled students, it is important to take into consideration the specific disabilities of the child. For example, students with more severe cognitive impairments may lack age-appropriate social understanding of complex interactions. Language impaired students may have appropriate understanding of social situations but may have difficulty communicating effectively with others. Other students may have an adequate repertoire of problem-solving behaviors but lack the opportunity to practice them because of the self-contained nature of their educational program. Prior to implementing a social problem-solving program, a thorough evaluation of the strengths and weaknesses of each student will enable the teacher to adapt the program and to be prepared to meet the needs of each child. (Some tools to assist in this are described in Chapter 9.) It may be advantageous to have heterogeneous groups when doing social problem solving and decision making so that children can learn from each other.

The resource center or other pullout program (supplemental instruction, group counseling) has the advantage of being a small group in a protected setting. This allows for a degree of intimacy and sharing not necessarily found in a larger class. In addition, because the resource center teacher provides a great deal of individual attention to each child, there may be a greater degree of trust and cohesion. It is important for the teacher to use this situation to advantage while keeping in mind that the goal of the social problem-solving and decision-making program is to enable students to function independently outside of the classroom. These settings can be special places to share problem-solving successes and challenges, review situations with the Problem Tracker, or sit down and work through a problem with the Student Conflict Manager.

It is usually relatively easy to implement social decision-making training in self-contained special education classes. The need for this program tends to be clear and the class usually has the flexibility to implement it without too much disruption in the schedule. Also, one is dealing with a group of students that stays together for a significant period of time with numerous opportunities to practice the skills in vivo. However, when working with self-contained classes, additional efforts must be made to ensure the generalization of these skills beyond the self-contained class. The goal of special education should be to teach students to compensate for their disabilities in order to function within the mainstream. If generalization is not specifically planned for in social skills, it will not occur.

Regularity

Establish a regular time and place for social problem-solving and decision-making activities. Convey to students that this is a special part of the week during which you will help them develop social skills and solve social problems. Giving this time a specific name such as the Sharing Circle (see p. 42) or "sharing time" and having the students form a circle or other special seating pattern can help to define this as different from the students' other educational activities.

FIG TESPN was initially developed as an alternative to presenting the problem-solving process as discrete steps. The theory behind this is that learning disabled students often have difficulty processing information in a sequential or linear manner. However, some learning disabled students will have difficulty integrating all the parts of the process together. Teachers should focus on both presenting FIG TESPN as a complete process and breaking down the process into discrete skills that can be taught individually. This can be done by repetition of the overall process during every lesson with a focus on one aspect of the process for in-depth understanding and practice.

Multisensory Varied Instructional Approaches

As with any other instructional material for learning disabled students, it is helpful to use a multisensory approach. Some students will benefit from a verbal presentation and discussion, others require visual stimuli and visual cues, and all students profit from actual practice of the skills through in-class role plays and homework assignments to use the skills outside of class. Other means of utilizing a multisensory approach include having students make a videotape (some can write the script, direct, or act), draw cartoons depicting FIG TESPN helping them solve a problem, and cut out pictures from magazines reflecting different feelings. In addition, popular television shows can be used as a stimulus for discussion with alternate endings developed by the students.

Although written assignments involving social problem solving can be helpful, this is often an aversive situation for students and should be kept to a minimum. Worksheets with guided questions requiring minimal written responses can be used. Also, teacher-developed checklists can both help students develop a better problem-solving vocabulary and reinforce the skills in a nonaversive manner. (Children often enjoy learning new words in a social problem-solving context because the words have relevance to them and also they will not be tested on the material.) For example, the teacher can read a story and the students can complete a worksheet such as the following:

1. In the story, how was Tommy feeling when his friends went to the movies without him?

    Tommy was feeling: (Circle how Tommy was feeling.)

    sad   lonely   rejected   happy   bored   tired   content

2. Did Tommy have a problem? If so, what was it?

    (Circle Tommy's problem.)

    Tommy did not have a problem.

    Tommy did not have any friends.

    Tommy did not communicate to his friends what he wanted.

    Tommy's friends are mean.

3. What was Tommy's goal? What did he want to have happen?

This approach can be adapted as described in the basic and extended Book Talk and literature analysis formats in Chapter 7.

Programs for the Gifted and Talented

At another extreme in terms of cognitive ability, but not necessarily in terms of social awareness, are students who display advanced abilities in some area of academic or creative talent. These students' social needs often are overlooked because their social sophistication is assumed to be commensurate with their intelligence. Obviously, this is not necessarily the case.

When working with gifted students, the similarities between the social problem-solving process and the scientific method can be pointed out. With older students, the connection to FIG TESPN as a mnemonic for the scientific method might be more appealing than presenting FIG TESPN as a character that helps them problem solve. FIG TESPN also can be discussed as an abstract process that can be applied to a variety of situations and problems.

With most programs, the social applications of social problem solving and decision making will be introduced prior to the academic applications. Teachers may wish to reverse this order for gifted students. They may be more comfortable with an initial use of social problem solving and decision making in an academic setting. They can then see how the same kind of problem solving can be applied to social problems as well.

When working on social problem-solving and decision-making activities, gifted students may have a broad "feelings" vocabulary and be able to list a variety of feelings; this does not mean that they can adequately differentiate these feelings in themselves or others or that they are aware of these feelings as they experience them in everyday interpersonal situations, especially stressful ones. Learning their Feelings Fingerprints is especially important for these children; further, an emphasis on awareness of feelings may help them explore new ways of knowing.

Gifted students tend to do well at brainstorming behavioral alternatives and anticipating consequences. It will be necessary to focus on practicing and role playing so that they will become comfortable *actually using the skills involved.* With all populations, it is necessary always to bring the discussion down to a concrete level and have them practice solving problems, either through behavioral rehearsal, in vivo classroom experiences, or assignments in which they monitor their behavior using the Problem Tracker. A cognitive understanding and ability to verbalize appropriate problem solving does not guarantee that they will exercise these skills spontaneously.

Reducing Perfectionism and Increasing Frustration Tolerance

Another aspect of gifted children sometimes overlooked because of their intelligence is a tendency to be perfectionistic and ironically to have a low frustration tolerance despite their high level of ability. In this case, the thoughts and feelings children have about their ability to succeed can interfere in their use of social problem-solving and decision-making skills. Addressing these negative self-statements is beyond the scope of this book; however, the teacher should be alert to these kinds of issues, especially if, despite a good plan, the student seems unable to carry it out.

One way of emphasizing the point that no one is perfect, and to reinforce the step of envisioning outcomes for each option, is to have a social studies lesson on "Great Mistakes in History." This unit can cover such topics as the rejection of Galileo's ideas concerning the orbit of the earth around the Sun, Columbus' voyage, Napoleon at Waterloo, the incorporation of slavery into the Constitution of the United States, the United States' treatment of Native Americans and the development of the system of Indian Reservations, the stock market crash of 1929 and the subsequent Great Depression, the appeasement of Germany following World

War I, the failure to act on information relating to treatment of the Japanese in America or the Jews in Europe during World War II, Hitler's invasion of Russia, the dropping of the first and/or second atomic bombs on Japan, Russia's decision to move missiles into Cuba, the "Bay of Pigs" attempted invasion of Cuba, the creation and production of the Edsel, Watergate, China's attempts to squelch democracy, Saddam Hussein's invasion of Kuwait that precipitated the Gulf War in 1992 and related conflicts, the Challenger Shuttle tragedy, the Hubble telescope, the baseball and hockey strikes of 1993, and scheduling classes before 8:30 A.M.

Note that these topics vary in seriousness and historical significance and that, for many of these topics, as well as others you might choose, there is some disagreement as to whether a mistake was in fact made, or what the nature of the mistake was. These variations can be presented to students, along with the request that they use the activity to help formulate (and justify) their opinion as to whether the event should be on your "mistakes" list next year.

Keep in mind that the purpose of this lesson is for children to see that everyone makes mistakes, even great leaders and scientists. Students can discuss or write about what unforeseen outcomes occurred as a result of the options chosen. They can then generate other options that could have been tried and imagine what potential outcomes might have arisen from them. This lesson can also be used with current events articles from the newspaper. The assignment is to find an article about a "mistake" that someone made and what outcomes were not envisioned by the participants. Students can then write other options and possible outcomes for the participants.

Finally, there are specific types of problems that gifted children encounter that may be useful to address. These topics include the following:

1. Social rejection and teasing from peers
2. Difficulty relating to peers due to a lack of shared interests
3. Pressures
4. Difficulty reading subtle social cues
5. "Eccentric" behavior that contributes to social rejection

Children with Attention-Deficit/Hyperactivity Disorder

If you have ever worked with children who have attention-deficit/hyperactivity disorder (ADHD) (or ADD, as it used to be called), you are aware of their deficits in social skills and their tendency to act impulsively, rather than make careful decisions. When working one to one, these children are often able to verbalize appropriate behaviors and are aware of consequences, but they seem oblivious to rules and repercussions when on their own. This can be frustrating to the teacher and to other students in the class. Ultimately, it is also frustrating to the child because of the inordinate amount of negative feedback he/she receives from others. Nevertheless, this child frequently finds her- or himself in trouble, but is unaware of how he/she got there.

Children with ADHD need to focus on the readiness skills, especially Keep Calm. This skill needs to be prompted and practiced frequently. It is a prerequisite skill because if students do not first stop their activity and become ready to attend to the problem, they will not be able to use the other, more complex skills of social problem solving and decision making. For those children having difficulty with Keep Calm, the Problem Tracker and Student Conflict Manager can be of value in helping them keep track of those situations that repeatedly provide them with their greatest self-control and attentional challenges.

The use of self-verbalization has been found to be effective in getting children to inhibit their impulsivity. The use of self-verbalization is implicit in FIG TESPN but needs to be made explicit for children with ADHD. Towards this end, the teacher should model the use of FIG TESPN frequently. The teacher should have students verbalize the steps as well as their responses. A fading procedure can be used where eventually the steps are whispered and then said silently to themselves. After all the steps have been taught and reinforced, the procedure can be shortened somewhat with a focus on the problem, potential solutions, planning the implementation of the solution, and self-feedback on the success of the plan. Self-prompts to stay focused on the problem can also be included. Programs for teaching self-verbalization (e.g., Braswell, 1993; Kendall, 1988) are compatible with FIG TESPN and can be used as an adjunct.

Another consideration for children with ADHD—especially if there is difficulty in using Keep Calm—is training them to use their feelings as a cue to problem solve. These children tend to use feelings as a cue to engage in an inappropriate behavior. The teacher will often have opportunities in the classroom to practice this. It requires the teacher to be alert to situations that can engender reactions in the child and then help the child use FIG TESPN prior to acting.

Assuming no other cognitive deficits, children with ADHD can often generate the problem, goal, and so forth. They then get stuck when required to carry out the plan. They may be able to create a plan but on follow-up have not carried it out. The teacher will need to break down the plan into units and monitor and reinforce each unit until the plan is carried out.

In general, children with ADHD respond well to frequent monitoring and feedback on their behavior. Formal monitoring and reinforcement procedures (as used in behavior modification programs) can be applied to the use of social problem-solving skills. For example, the teacher can have a chart on which use of Keep Calm and FIG TESPN are monitored. Each spontaneous use earns one point. Five points entitles the student to a specific reward such as free time or, getting help from an older student with their homework. The teacher may also wish to include the student's self-report of use of a social problem-solving and decision-making technique. Although the teacher cannot verify the report, it encourages the student to at least think of times outside the classroom when they could have used it.

Those working with students who have ADHD or related problems will find *Meeting the ADD Challenge* (Gordon & Asher, 1994) to be an invaluable guide with clear, practical suggestions that are fully compatible with the approaches described herein.

Emotionally Disturbed Populations

Emotionally disturbed (ED) populations are among the most challenging and the most needy in terms of teaching social skills. Their inclusion in mainstream classrooms has become a source of vexation for many teachers, school practitioners, and administrators, in part because the challenges and preparations needed for this combination tend not to be given adequate sustained attention. Although it is beyond the scope of this book to provide comprehensive solutions to these concerns, there are several facets of the issue that, when clarified, can increase the chances of successful work with the ED population.

With this population, it is important to differentiate between those with a skill deficit and those with a performance deficit. Skill deficit means that students have not mastered the basic social skills necessary to engage appropriately with others or solve social problems. Performance deficit means that students have the skills but do not use them due to a lack of intrinsic or extrinsic motivators. With the former group, there needs to be an emphasis on skill development. With the latter group, it is necessary to identify the motivators. Sometimes these motivators can be reframed in such a way as to encourage the ED student to use social problem-solving and decision-making skills. You do not help the child become a better thief if money is their motivation, but you can help the child become aware of the consequences of that solution and generate behavioral alternatives for reaching their goal of getting money. It may also be necessary to establish motivators in the program, that is, the consequences for inappropriate social behaviors at school are aversive and the consequences for prosocial behaviors and the use of social problem solving and decision making are desirable.

With an ED population, there are obviously issues in addition to social skills that interfere in social development. However, social skills pro-motion can help the children break out of maladaptive behavior patterns and begin to feel more capable. These children may assume that regard-less of their behaviors, the outcomes will be negative. Further, time must be spent acknowledging their strengths and helping them to see that they have contributions to make to their classrooms and schools (Brendtro et al., 1991). Specific social problem-solving and decision-making lessons have been developed that focus on the critical area of "put-downs" and positive esteem builders in ED populations (Hett & Clabby, 1993). It is im-portant to provide small successes for them so they can begin to see the usefulness of appropriate social skills in enabling them to have their needs met and for them to begin to experience the naturally reinforcing conse-quences of appropriate social behavior.

With these fragile children, it is also necessary to "inoculate" them against further experiences of failure and rejection. In the planning phase, it is essential to anticipate potential obstacles to implementing their plan and achieving their goal. Once these obstacles have been identified, sec-ond-order FIG TESPNs can be done to solve these problems, as described in Chapter 4. Also, the child must be taught and reinforced for self-coping statements when confronted with challenges. The last step, "Now what?," can also include teaching of and prompting for self-coping statements.

Finally, the modality of video-based lessons, especially those using TVDRP and other approaches described in Chapter 5, are powerful sources of successful learning for ED students. This is in part because chil-dren with emotional problems often suffer from low self-esteem. They are particularly concerned with acting "cool" (or whatever the current term might be!). Admitting to a problem can be threatening, as it might dimin-ish what they perceive as their "status." Of course, these kinds of process-es operate in all children; but among ED populations, it is central to their view of self, thus their tolerance of ridicule, shame, or embarrassment is low and their reactions are correspondingly intense. Video modalities in-troduce the buffer of hypothetical situations so that neither they nor the other children with whom they might be working have to personalize the issues involved. Much can be worked out using the characters in the video and their problems. In recognition of the power of video modalities (as well as the use of computers), the journal *Teaching Exceptional Children* de-voted a special issue ("Using Videotape Technology," 1995) to this topic, including many specific school-tested intervention ideas, in spring 1995.

Children of Difference

With increasingly pluralistic, multicultural, and ethnically diverse school populations, educators will constantly face children who are different than the majority group in their classrooms, schools, and/or communities. In this section, rather than addressing every other subpopulation with whom school professionals might find themselves working, guidelines will be provided on how to adapt the program to meet the needs of any "population of difference." By focusing on the concepts of differentness, strengths, respect for diversity, and the following principles, a social decision making program can be adapted to diverse populations such as ethnic minorities, children of poverty, children of alcoholics, children of divorce, or underachievers.

1. *Identify the strengths of the population and use the strengths to bolster self-esteem and compensate for areas of weakness.* For example, children who have experienced stress due to family or environmental problems can discuss how they have successfully coped with these problems in the past. These successful problem-solving examples can be put into the FIG TESPN framework. Because of their experiences, some students may have strengths in sensitivity toward feelings, although they might not be dealing with these feelings appropriately.

2. *Identify specific needs of the population in terms of knowledge, skill, or attitude.* For example, in a program for teen-age pregnancy prevention, it will be necessary to inform students about what is actually involved in raising a child so that they will be able to "envision the end results" more accurately. Some populations will need more skill development than others in effective communication skills. Additional activities can be developed around these needs.

3. *Review the readiness skills and FIG TESPN and identify those skills that may be most readily mastered and those that may be most difficult.* This will give the school practitioner an indication of the pace at which to work. Each lesson can last one session or be continued through several lessons. Also, lessons can be repeated or extended. Repetition is necessary for mastery. The overall age and level of cognitive development will also influence the pace and concreteness of the lessons.

4. *Identify typical problems the children face and tailor instruction to those problems.* You may first wish to use more general, less threatening examples and then move to more personal and relevant ones. Stories that provide analogous situations are useful.

5. *Be sensitive to the differences that these children have in terms of perspective and social norms.* Cultural and social factors influence the goals and potential solutions that will be generated. Regardless of the population the teacher is working with, it is necessary for the teacher to suspend critical judgment of anything proposed by the student. The teacher's role is to facilitate thinking through the problem so that better decisions can be made

by the child. If the teacher censors certain goals or options, this puts the teacher in an authority role and inhibits the children's ability to think through to the consequences of their actions.

6. *Review the steps in FIG TESPN and identify those steps that may be most important to the population.* Emphasize those steps through extended discussion or lessons to address them. For example, for children with a substance abuse problem, it will be important to focus on their goals. What do they want out of life? Where would they like to be in 5 years? Then, focus on end results. If they continue to use drugs, where will they be in 5 years? With children of divorce, extra attention to clarifying feelings will be important.

Above all, when tailoring the program to a subgroup, it is necessary for the teacher or other group leader to listen to the children. Through active listening, the students will feel that their experiences are validated and accepted. In addition, the teacher can then begin to identify the specific circumstances, strengths, and needs of the children. Through listening, teachers can be sensitive to students and can adapt the lessons to the students' needs. A concise overview and guidelines for carrying out these types of interventions can be found in Zins and Elias (1993).

GENERAL PRINCIPLES OF CONSULTATION BY SCHOOL PRACTITIONERS

Note that the role of the school practitioner is largely that of a consultant and catalyst. Guidance counselors, school psychologists and social workers, learning specialists, substance awareness coordinators, school nurses and health educators, and other school practitioners, by virtue of their many responsibilities and the fact they there are relatively few of them, must work in ways that teach and empower others who have more direct contact time with students. This, in essence, requires skills in functioning in a consultative role. Although this may be familiar, generally the role involves what is known as "case-centered consultation," which revolves around one student. Yet, given the enormity of the needs described earlier and the flexibility and expertise of many school practitioners, working at the group, classroom, and school levels is virtually a necessity. Such work can be extremely rewarding—though not without its challenges, trepidations, and frustrations—and places the school practitioner at the front lines of efforts to build student health and social competence in lasting, systemic ways, thereby helping to prevent a range of problem behaviors that would be more likely to result without such intervention.

Develop Pilot Programs

The first principle of change in an organizational setting is to start small. It is recommended that all efforts in social decision-making program implementation be called "pilot" programs. This accomplishes two things. One, it establishes appropriate expectations on everyone's part. Social decision-making programs *are* out to change the world, but this goal can only be achieved one child at a time, one situation at a time. All those involved in the program either actively (delivering services) or passively (sanctioning the program, such as administrators and parents) need to understand that this is a long-range project because extremely complex skills are being taught. One would not expect a remedial reading class to read Shakespeare by the end of the year nor should one expect a social skills class to produce independent problem solvers after one year of implementation. Collecting outcome data is important for improving the program and verifying its effects (see Chapter 9) but initial expectations should be modest and realistic.

The second reason for calling the initial effort a pilot project is that it helps protect the program from failure. Pilot programs are allowed to fail because they are learning experiences for all involved. When a pilot program is started, it is not touted as "THE ANSWER." Pilot programs are a good place to begin, get some experience, see how the program works or does not work in the setting, and make some adaptations before the "real" program is implemented. It is reasonable to expect that a successful program will take from 3 to 5 years to develop.

In keeping with the limited pilot nature of the initial program, the consultant should decide where, what, how, and with whom the program should be started. Often special education programs are the most receptive because the need is most obvious and they have the flexibility in scheduling. But anywhere a need has been identified is a good place to start. For example, sometimes due to the mix of students, a particular classroom is experiencing social difficulties. Or, perhaps a vocal group of parents have expressed a need for guidance in helping their children develop better problem-solving skills. Drug awareness and family life programs are also good places to start.

When deciding "what" to start with, again, start small. One advantage of the FIG TESPN program is that it can be started anywhere. Although it is usually best to start with readiness activities such as Keep Calm and BEST, one can also get the program started by using academic applications. In addition, FIG TESPN can be used as a systematic long-term program or as a crisis intervention tool. Once the need and point of entry have been established, what material can be covered will usually become apparent.

It is helpful for consultants to remember that they also are salespersons. Pulling out a particular worksheet or activity and discussing it with a teacher to address a specific problem may be a way of getting the foot in the door. If this is received positively, then additional program elements can be introduced.

Some sales are easier than others. Some parents, teachers, and administrators will approach the consultant looking for a social skills program. Others must first be convinced of the need to address the social and emotional aspects of learning. When piloting the program, it is best to start with those already sold on the program. Successful implementation requires ownership by both the implementers and the children receiving the program. Therefore, even with those sold already, the new program should be adapted to make it consistent with their current program and style of teaching. Once a successful program is running, others can see it, and the leaders running it can give testimonials as to its effectiveness. This will be the best way to advertise a program and help it expand as you think appropriate.

Readiness for Consultation and Program Development

Prior to training others to implement the program, it is useful to determine readiness for consultation. The first step is to establish a relationship with the consultee that is based on mutual professional respect. When beginning a consultation process, the "fit" between consultant and consultee must be assessed. Some relationships are easier to build than others depending on factors such as personality, professional experience and knowledge, perceived need for consultation service, organizational sanctions and inhibitions, and prior experiences both as a consultant and consultee.

Getting Started: The Hardest Task

There are basically two ways for consultants to get a program going. One is to do it themselves, with others peripherally involved; the other is to identify specific staff members to train and deliver the program. Our preference is to train others from the start. It sets an empowering tone and conveys professional respect. It builds on local resources and makes a statement that local continuity is the essential ingredient in the program's long-term success (i.e., it's what _you_ can do that matters, not what the outside visitor can do). Finally, it is cost effective for a consultant to work with a number of other professionals, and it also builds local expertise and a common knowledge base. Certainly, it is important for implementers to have some kind of vision of what the program looks like when it is carried out; but there are videos available, lessons by other professionals in other sites that can be observed, and "mock" or "demonstration" activities that can be arranged (Bruene-Butler, Schuyler, & Clabby, 1993).

Once the where, what, who, and when have been identified, "how" to implement a social decision-making program looms as the next challenge. But, once consultants are familiar with the social problem-solving and decision-making process, the answer should become obvious. First, consultants should Keep Calm; then, using their BEST communication skills, they should assess what the staff members' Feelings are about children's social difficulties. Specific types of Problems that the children are having can then be identified, the purpose of which is to establish Goals for the program. In conjunction with the staff members identified for involvement, different Things to do should be generated. Here, it is important to consider options that are consistent with the individual's circumstances and style of teaching. For example, an academically oriented teacher may be more comfortable with starting with academic applications or introducing Keep Calm as a strategy for relieving test anxiety.

After Outcomes are envisioned, a good way to start can be Selected. Again, the emphasis is on the pilot nature of the first year. It is important to anticipate obstacles to the program, such as time constraints, parental objection, skill deficits in both staff and children, videotape player availability, computer access, and lag time in ordering materials. The greater the degree to which Planning is done with the staff members involved, the better chance that the program will be implemented as planned.

For the consultant, the last step, "Notice what happened and now what," is extremely important. Ongoing monitoring and consultation will be necessary in order to ensure success. The consultant should plan on sitting in on sessions and meeting with staff on a regular basis to review the program and its implementation. Formal and informal tools for planning, monitoring, and evaluating programs are presented in Chapter 9.

Handling Glitches

Occasionally, a leader of a social problem-solving group will get stuck. Students may not be "buying into" the program or the leader may have difficulty using the facilitative approach. When this occurs, it can be helpful for the leader to observe someone else facilitating a group. This can be another staff member, someone in another setting, or, if necessary, the consultant, serving as a co-leader. It is also helpful to have others observe the group and provide feedback in a nonthreatening manner. This is especially helpful when done in a group supervision context (see below).

After the program is in place, it will be time to begin to promote generalization. This can be done by expanding the program into other areas of the children's day. Other staff members should be trained in using the prompts to remind children of the skills learned in the social decision-making program. In a school setting, it is especially important to train lunch aides and teachers of special subjects (art, music, gym) to use the specific prompts. Another way of promoting generalization is to use the Problem Trackers in other settings that are then brought back to the instructional setting so that there can be a discussion of how to make the ideas work, for example, in the lunchroom or on the bus.

Group Supervision

Although implementing a social skills training program in schools often involves an outside consultant or trained consultant within the district, after the program is in place with supplementary curriculum materials, local implementers should begin to recognize the expertise they have to carry on and further develop the program. A group supervision program among school practitioners using social problem solving can provide the additional support, program development, and program refinement necessary to maximize the program's effectiveness.

Group supervision assumes a certain level of knowledge and skill. Prior to beginning, it would be helpful for all implementers to be familiar with this book or some other common source of related social problem-solving and decision-making instructional information. In addition, they should be prepared to work on social skills and decision making on a regular and frequent basis with the students. A set of formal plans is helpful, but not essential; however, it is necessary for implementers to have documented their activities in some manner, such as through the use of Feedback Sheets (Chapter 9).

The goals of the group supervision are:

1. To assist implementers in planning their social problem-solving and decision-making activities
2. To assist implementers in working through individual problems with the social problem-solving and decision-making activities
3. To assist implementers in working with individual students who are experiencing problems in social and/or academic areas
4. To build a library of supplementary curriculum/activity materials
5. To further adapt and develop the entire social problem-solving and decision-making approach as used in one's setting

It is important for the group to meet on a regular and relatively frequent basis. The meeting schedule should be established in the beginning of the year. At the beginning of each session, an agenda should be developed. We have found the following framework to be useful.

1. Review of social problem-solving and decision-making activities or lessons taught and problems/successes encountered
2. Sharing of sample materials, lessons, and worksheets developed by individual teachers (copies for all participants should be brought)
3. Brainstorming and initial outlining of additional lessons designed to meet specific classroom needs
4. Individual problems, either in terms of lessons or students

During the group supervision, it is important to stay on topic and proceed in an organized manner. Although some informal information exchange may be helpful, this should be kept to a minimum. A certain amount of time can be allotted to this on the agenda. (Things will go most smoothly if all implementers are at least somewhat familiar with the program and/or curriculum materials that others are using. One or two initial meetings might be devoted to building this common knowledge base.) Although group supervision is leaderless, there should be a rotating "facilitator" whose responsibility is to keep the discussion on topic, to coordinate any additional actions that are planned during the meeting, and to see to the logistics for the meetings (agenda, time, space, refreshments, materials).

The last several group supervision meetings of the school year should be dedicated to evaluating the year's social decision-making and problem-solving activities and solidifying plans for the following year. This should include evaluating the curriculum and related activities, how they were implemented, and the group supervision process. For these meetings, group members may wish to come to the meeting with the following:

1. The best lessons and activities and why
2. The worst lessons and activities and why
3. Implementation successes
4. Implementation failures
5. Ratings (using scales devised earlier by the group) on the group supervision and suggestions on how to improve it
6. Personal and general ideas/plans for the following year's social problem-solving and decision-making activities and their implementation

In addition to group supervision, or when group supervision is not feasible, there will be times when it is useful to tap some external experience and expertise in social decision-making instruction. Having recognized this issue throughout the course of our work, several "antidotes for isolation" are available as follows:

♦ Professional development/continuing education workshops provide an ongoing opportunity for skill advancement. Based at such places as the Center for Applied Psychology at Rutgers University, people gather to share in-training experiences, which also leads to networks of sustained informal contacts.

♦ On-site national training brings the social problem-solving approach to local groups through the NDN. Facilitators in each U.S. state and territory serve as a network to help those in public and private schools access relevant programs that have been approved by the Program Effectiveness Panel of the U.S. Department of Education.

♦ Newsletters, such as the *The Problem Solving Connection Newsletter (PSC)*, published by the Social Problem Solving Unit of the University of Medicine and Dentistry of New Jersey—Community Mental Health Center (UMDNJ-CMHC) at Piscataway, serve as means of sharing instructional and programmatic innovations, triumphs, problems, and questions. The *PSC* is sent two or three times per year to hundreds of educators around the country as well as in the United Kingdom, Australia, and Canada, who are interested in or are actively using social problem solving and related approaches. Such newsletters are best designed as resource exchanges. In future years, as e-mail and other forms of electronic networking become more commonly used and more easily accessible, such networking will go "on line" to make advice giving and receiving more current.

♦ Training centers, such as those established at UMDNJ-CMHC at Piscataway, which has a service delivery unit called the Social Problem Solving Unit, and at the Consultation Center at Yale University Medical School, provide phone-in services through which questions are answered by a consultant, send faxes of existing informational and instructional materials and documents with which one might not be familiar, and arrange for trainings.

INVOLVING PARENTS: THE CHALLENGE AND THE OPPORTUNITY

A social decision-making program is enriched by finding meaningful roles for parents. This is as true at the high school level as it is earlier; however, it is recognized that the earlier parents find roles in this (or any) element of schooling, the more likely they are to sustain those roles. There are three levels at which parents can be engaged in a social decision-making program: they can be *informed, involved,* or *included.*

♦ *Informing* parents means letting them know what is going on in the classroom. This can occur at back-to-school nights or special parent meetings by describing the program or, most effectively, by running groups of parents through a simulated lesson. Several meetings over the course of the year can be held, corresponding to different phases of social decision making instruction.

♦ *Involving* parents means that one seeks their active support of the school-based learning and/or home extensions of that learning. This can occur through meetings but also through what our colleague Charlotte Hett calls "refrigerator notes." These are one-page handouts that summarize a concept taught in class (e.g., Classroom Constitution, Keep Calm, FIG TESPN) and make concrete suggestions to parents about how they can recognize and reinforce the use of the skill by the child, use prompts and cues to elicit the skill in Trigger Situations, and/or apply the skill to commonly recurring home situations and routines.

♦ *Including* parents means that parents are given the skills to creatively integrate social decision making into their home routines and parenting practices. This can occur by having them read relevant resource materials (see Appendix B) or by having four to six session group meetings, co-led by teachers and/or school psychologists, social workers, guidance counselors, health educators, or other interested school practitioners. A useful framework for such sessions is to have group members read specific reading material and discuss uses of the ideas and methods with children from preschool through high school as relevant to a particular group, ways parents can use the skills to relieve their own life stress, and application of the ideas to various topics such as homework, discipline, peer relationships, and college and career choices. Parenting centers can be developed and staffed, at least in part, by parents to gather and provide parenting information, using methods such as those suggested for group supervision to compile parent questions and suggested solutions to problems.

Materials exist in support of these options. Hett and Krikorian (1993) describe how to create parent newsletters and other forms of parental involvement. Clabby and Elias (1986) and Shure (1994) provide practical translations of school-based social problem solving into ideas and anecdotes easily used by parents; Shure's work is focused especially on younger children. Also available is computer software that brings the social problem-solving process into the home, for use by parents and families (Psychological Enterprises Incorporated, 1993). Elias and Clabby (1992) provide a step-by-step outline of how to engage parents in initial meetings concerning social problem-solving activities to which their children are being exposed. Grady, Kline, Belanoff, and Snow (1993) provide outstanding materials for working with groups of parents of students of middle school or high school age.

CHAPTER 9

Practical Tools for Assessment: Monitoring Intervention Implementation and Impact

♦

> There are times when we cannot let other people do our thinking
> for us; we must think for ourselves. And we must learn to think for
> ourselves. . . . The point is that students must be encouraged to
> become reasonable for their own good (i.e., as a step toward their
> own autonomy) and not just for our good (i.e., because the
> growing rationalization of the society requires it).
> —*Lipman (1988, p. 43)*

There always is a gap between reading about new interventions, curriculum, and instruction procedures and putting them into action. At times, that gap can widen into an impassable chasm, according to those who study the implementation of innovations into existing systems. However, there are certain things that can be done to ensure that the gap remains small, and eventually disappears. The previous chapter discussed ways of tailoring programs and of maintaining ongoing consultation and quality control. This chapter focuses on the role of monitoring and evaluation in keeping track of one's goals for a program and the extent to which they are being achieved.

THE PROGRAM/INTERVENTION LIFE CYCLE

Much has been written about the "life" of programs in schools, including quite a bit that relates specifically to programs in the social and affective domain (Basch, 1983; Elias & Clabby, 1992; Fullan, 1993; Huberman & Miles, 1984; Sarason, 1982; Weissberg, 1985). In contemplating the monitoring of implementation and impact, it can be helpful to have a vision of the road upon which one is embarking.

The Pilot Stage: Start Things Off and Keep Them Going

The history of school change—both large scale and classroom-sized—shows that change begins with a small pilot effort. This is equally true for lasting, meaningful change in curriculum and instruction procedures. Select some aspect of what you have read in the preceding chapters and set up a pilot project in which you begin to apply the ideas and monitor how well they work. Set very modest goals; do not begin a program by expecting the program to be the instrument to solve your most difficult classroom or behavioral problems.

The history of school change shows that successful program development takes anywhere from 3 to 5 years. The pilot year provides the implementer with the basic idea of how the procedure works. It is a significant step to go from reading about a program to actually putting it into practice. After the first-year pilot activities, the implementer is in a much better position to think about how the program really works and how it can apply to his or her own particular concerns. Further, a pilot year, by its very nature, should contain various different approaches to carrying out the program; there should be an experimental spirit. One might try for example, using social decision making by first attempting to work with one or two self-control and social awareness skills. Or, one might find that one would like to begin by applying FIG TESPN to social studies or language arts. Perhaps one would begin by instituting a weekly ½-hour period when the class will meet for group sharing and discussion, and proceed using the type of framework outlined in Chapters 3 and 4. The point is that in year 1 several different things should be attempted so as to ascertain their "fit."

The analogy of being in a marvelous clothing store and taking some time to try on different things is quite appropriate here. Similar to being in a clothing store, one will find that one begins to narrow down the outfits with which one is most comfortable. And, once again like the clothing store, one may choose to purchase one or many outfits, depending on one's particular situation. Indeed, seasons change. Applications of social decision making that are successful at one particular time with one particular grade level or student population may evolve as one continues to work with that population, or may shift radically as one encounters a new "season." The second year, therefore, is devoted to selecting those outfits with which one is most pleased, putting them into one's wardrobe throughout the entire year, and then seeing how one's life is affected by their presence.

The first year is a familiarization year; the second year is the year for the instructor to master what he or she is attempting to do. The third year is what is most often referred to as the consolidation year (Elias & Clabby, 1992). This is the year in which one has mastered the instructional procedures to the point where one is now prepared to do one's best work with them. By the third year, and sometimes through the course of a fourth and fifth year, the procedures are being mastered and the children become the beneficiaries of highly competent instruction.

The Consolidation Stage: Be Prepared for Changes in Roles

A new program is not simply a set of activities. It requires integration into one's view of one's role in the schools. The social problem-solving approach is aligned with several different kinds of roles. When using this approach, educators become significant *sources of support*, by providing a positive, caring, safe, predictable learning environment. By focusing on self-control and social awareness, educators make it clear that there is a structure and set of limits that will be respected, and that the feelings and rights of other people are included in that "safe area." Another role is that of a *facilitator of others' thinking* through the use of FIG TESPN and facilitative questioning and modeling techniques. Instructors let it be known that they value students' thoughtfulness. They convey the fact that their role is not to solve children's problems but to give the children the skills to solve their own problems. Along with this role is an expectation that children *can* solve their own problems; this is a great motivator and encourager particularly for children with learning difficulties or a history of disengagement from the school. An additional role is as the *prompter of self-control and social awareness*. Social problem-solving interventions operate based on an implicit, shared responsibility for learning. Instructors provide concepts, and then seek to help students to understand their appropriate use by prompting the use of the relevant skills as needed. Finally, the instructor takes on the role of *provider of thinking frameworks*. Many of the activities in Chapters 3, 4, 5, and 6 are alternative ways of building children's thoughtful social decision making and problem solving. These frameworks are applied to social studies, to monitoring one's own progress, to behavioral interactions with peers, and to a variety of other areas. They serve as road maps for children on the ultimate road to academic and social success and health.

These variations in role pervade one's interactions with students, extending well beyond the specific instructional time in which new procedures are being used. It is for this reason that we emphasize the importance of classroom teachers carrying out social decision-making activities, rather than having such activities conveyed primarily through pullout programs or by having professionals come into the classroom on a weekly basis and work with the students.

TRACKING PROGRAM PROGRESS: THE CONTRACTED EVALUATION PLAN WORKSHEET

The life cycle of programs provides a framework for determining when certain types of goals become salient, as well the timing around which to look for their appearance. An important component of any social problem-solving program is measuring the impact the instruction is having on its recipients. A multifaceted approach that enables one to gain a closer look at the benefits and problems that have occurred during the time a program has been implemented involves what is known as a "program evaluation study." The outcomes of an evaluation study are useful in many ways. The most obvious examples are (1) as an aid in modifying a program to better fit its recipients and (2) as a determining factor in decisions to continue or discontinue implementing a program.

An evaluation is most successful when carefully planned before any program implementation begins. Another way of saying this is that *evaluation should be thought of as part of a program and built in from the beginning.* The "Contracted Evaluation Plan (CEP) Worksheet" is a valuable aid in deciding what will be evaluated and how and in formulating an evaluation plan (Papke & Elias, 1993). Table 9.1 contains an outline of the CEP sequence of questions that should be answered prior to beginning any evaluation study, however minimal it may be. Further, the CEP serves as a clarifying tool for aspects of intervention planning and implementation.

The outline suggests that one begin with a basic description of the program to be studied. In a brief narrative, indicate the scope of the program, such as what and how many schools, teachers, and students are involved. Program goals, as well as whatever will occur as part of the program, also should be listed. There should be agreement about who will do the actual work with students and the timeline of the program for a given year.

The CEP then goes on to pose a series of decisions that must be made concerning the nature of the evaluation and, therefore, of the design of the intervention program. Always keep in mind the goals of the program in making these decisions. For example, pre- and posttesting for skill gain in a new program might be misleading. When implementers are newly trained and unfamiliar with the intervention procedures, consumer satisfaction (teacher and student) data indicating receptivity to the program and implementers' comfort in carrying out the procedures may be the highest priority.

TABLE 9.1. CEP Outline

Briefly describe program being evaluated.

Nature of evaluation—will your evaluation involve any of the following?
 a. Pretest–posttest
 b. Only a follow-up of work done during previous school year
 c. Gathering of baseline data
 d. Other (please explain)

What are the questions you want to answer? These questions should reflect your goals (i.e., process/implementation; skill gains/changes; relative changes; long-term outcomes).

What are the pretest instruments that you want to use?

When will the pretest instruments be administered?

Who will complete the pretest instruments?

Who will administer the pretest instruments? What procedures will be followed for administration of the pretest instruments?

How will the pretest data be analyzed or summarized? When is this information needed?

What are the posttest instruments that you want to use?

When will the posttest instruments be administered?

Who will complete the posttest instruments?

Who will administer the posttest instruments? What procedures will be followed for administration of the posttest instruments?

How will the posttest data be analyzed or summarized? When is this information needed?

When is the final report due? For whom is the report intended?

Who is going to be responsible for the write-up of the final report, to provide the feedback regarding the questions and instruments?

Note: All CEPs should include the name of district, classrooms, and so forth; the person evaluating program; and the date the Plan was completed. CEPs should be reviewed, commented on, and signed-off on by the supervisor or coordinator of the evaluation, the relevant principal or other administrator, and any person serving as a liaison to a relevant social decision-making, life skills, or other related school committee.

MONITORING THE PROCESS OF IMPLEMENTATION

Observation of Social Problem Solving

Interventions have key elements that must be in place to ensure that they maintain their integrity and are likely to have the effects one expects. For social problem-solving interventions, Table 9.2 presents a rating sheet that can be used for specific or global observation of social problem-solving activities. While sections 1 and 2 contain valuable group-leading informa-

TABLE 9.2. Techniques for Leading Social Decision-Making Discussions: Observational Checklist

Please complete this section before any observing or taping and self-rating.

Name and position of leader/facilitator: _____

Name and position of observer/rater: _____

Date of observation/rating: _____

Type of setting/topic of lesson (e.g., 23 fourth graders/review of Keep Calm): _____

Used	Used often	
		1. Elicits information
___	___	♦ Attends to verbal and nonverbal messages
___	___	♦ Reviews previous material
___	___	♦ Uses the "two-question rule" and follows a question with a question
___	___	♦ Allows waiting time after asking questions
___	___	♦ Clarifies comments and links to what others have said
		2. Provides supportive environment
___	___	♦ Uses inviting, varied voice tone; clear, well-paced speech
___	___	♦ Paraphrases children's responses and reflects feelings
___	___	♦ Accepts responses and asks for others
___	___	♦ Establishes clear rules (e.g., letting others speak without interrupting) and gives clear directions
___	___	♦ Praises before criticizing; gives positive, constructive feedback
___	___	♦ Praises, acknowledges participation
___	___	♦ Shows patience in responding to children's questions, confusions, off-task behavior
		3. Elicits thoughtful decision making and problem solving
___	___	♦ Uses prompts and cues (e.g., Keep Calm, FIG TESPN)
___	___	♦ Models own thinking and decision-making, own use of social decision making steps
___	___	♦ Provides a balance of open-ended asking, suggesting, and telling; guides and encourages thinking rather than being evaluative and providing "answers"
___	___	♦ Uses facilitative questioning techniques (open-ended; how, when, what else, what if, what might; Probe questions)
___	___	♦ Uses the Columbo technique
___	___	♦ Suggests use of self-control, social awareness, and social decision-making skills by students
___	___	♦ Encourages covert rehearsal (visualization, drawing, writing)
___	___	♦ Elicits linkages to students' own personal experiences; starts with hypotheticals and moves to actual situations

(continued)

TABLE 9.2 *(continued)*

Used	Used often	
		4. Encourages action
____	____	• Elicits details of specific planning; makes linkages to what will be done in the future
____	____	• Conducts behavioral rehearsal, guided practice
____	____	• Uses TVDRP

tion, sections 3 and 4 are more closely tailored to social problem solving. The rating can be completed via live observation or via a tape of the session, and consultants or teams of teachers can exchange information on ways to improve the delivery of the material.

Feedback on Implementation of Activities

Over the years of social problem-solving work, no tool has been of greater value than the Activity/Curriculum Feedback Sheet (Elias & Clabby, 1989; see outline in Table 9.3). The Feedback Sheet should be completed by implementers (and also by observers) after every activity or curriculum/instructional unit. The information captured is crucial for tailoring a program to a setting's unique needs. It provides a tangible reminder of

TABLE 9.3. Outline of Activity/Curriculum Feedback Sheet

Leader's name: _____

Date: _____

Class period(s)/activities/lessons conducted: _____

General outline of lesson or class activities:

Student reactions to this session (for whom was it most, least effective):

Most effective or favorable aspects of this session:

Least effective or favorable aspects of this session:

Describe implementation issues that required your attention:

Points to follow up in the next class meeting:

Suggested changes in this lesson/activity for the future:

where to pick up a subsequent activity after one stops for the day. For revision and future planning purposes, the Feedback Sheets serve as written records of how to improve the activity for the future. Considering all the information provided, the Feedback Sheet is as cost-efficient and user-friendly an implementation monitoring tool as we have seen.

Consumer Satisfaction

Regardless of the design of a program, the receptivity and responsiveness of the primary consumers of programs—the students and the implementers—must be examined. Table 9.4 contains an outline of a survey of students' opinions; it begins with a like/dislike dimension, moves to open-ended questions about the activities, and then follows with a variety of forced choice questions about different aspects of the program and their perceived use. Finally, students are asked to provide a brief vignette of a time they used the skills they were taught. Table 9.5 contains the same type of survey, except with a focus on implementer satisfaction.

TABLE 9.4. Outline of Student Satisfaction Survey

1. I thought the social problem-solving lessons were:
    lots of fun   pretty good   OK   no fun at all

2. I would like to have lessons like this:
    more often   just like we had them   once in a while   never again

3. What were the best things about the lessons?

4. What would make the lessons better?

5. These lessons have helped me to: [answer yes or no]
    get to know students in my class better
    handle my problems better
    feel happier
    stay calmer [others can be added as desired]

6. I use the things I learned in the lessons when I am: [answer yes or no]
    in class
    at lunch
    at gym
    in the hallway (between classes)
    at home, with my parents
    at home, with my brothers and sisters
    with my friends [others can be added as desired]

7. Please write about one or two times you used what you learned to help you with a problem at school or at home. Tell how you solved the problem and what was most helpful to you.

TABLE 9.5. Outline of Survey of Teacher/Implementer Opinions

I thought the lessons/activities were:
highly valuable   moderately valuable   of some value   of little value

I would like to continue using the program next year:
yes   no   unsure

What were the most valuable aspects of the program?

What difficulties were there in implementing the program?

I used the prompts and cues at times other than during the formal lesson:
often   sometimes   rarely   never

The lessons/activities have helped me to: [answer yes or no]
get to know my class/group better
manage classroom/group problems better
maintain a positive classroom atmosphere
increase students' social and emotional learning
other:

The lessons/activities helped the students in my class/group to:
[answer yes or no]
get to know each other better
handle their problems better
respect each others' differences
stay calmer
other:

In what situations did you see your students using the skills they were taught in the lessons/activities/group?

Please write about one or two times you and/or your students were able to use the skills in the lessons/activities to help with a problem. Tell how the problem was solved and how the skills covered were helpful.

Steer the Program toward Long-Term Success: Guidelines for Enduring Implementation Processes

School professionals who read about model programs in the literature often wonder, with good reason, how these programs manage in the real world of the schools, especially after the exciting start-up period is over. The School Intervention Implementation Study examined this question in a survey of over 550 operating school districts in New Jersey, ranging from urban to rural to suburban and even seashore districts (Elias, Gager, & Hancock, 1994). The study yielded several empirically derived guidelines that those interested in long-term program institutionalization with a high degree of fidelity to the original structure, goals, and purposes of the program might wish to consider (see Table 9.6.)

The guidelines are structured into two areas of consideration: aspects

TABLE 9.6. Guidelines for Successful Long-Term Implementation of Interventions

Aspects of implementation to encourage:

1. At first, the program should be implemented on a small or pilot scale.

2. At least one person or group in the district should serve as a strong advocate or champion for the program.

3. Persons carrying out the program must be committed to the program and believe it is an essential part of education in the community.

4. Persons who carry out the program need to share high morale, good communication, and a sense of ownership concerning the program.

5. There should be an ongoing process of formal and informal training of persons carrying out the program, involving such procedures as co-teaching, mutual observation, discussion and planning groups, or coaching.

6. The program materials are varied and actively engage learners.

7. The program's format allows it to complement and enhance other ongoing curricular areas.

8. The program engenders mutual respect and support among students.

9. There must be a regularly scheduled and adhered to time allotted for the program.

10. The program is appropriate for special education students.

11. Special education students must be regular recipients of the program; their schedules for pullout activities must be modified so as to not exclude them from social problem-solving activities.

12. Recipients should express satisfaction with the program.

13. There must be a program coordinator, facilitator, or committee that keeps track of the program and works to identify and resolve day-to-day problems.

14. Community individuals such as police, athletes, or business people can be coached to work effectively in the schools to help meet program goals, but must work in curricular and instructional harmony with those goals.

15. Persons who are new at carrying out the program should be trained by acknowledged expert trainers, whether from within the district or outside.

16. The program should be used in a systematic way throughout much, if not all, of the school district.

17. Once in place, programs that are "high profile"/high visibility in the school are more likely to be sustained.

Signs of problematic implementation about which to be wary; or, you should start to worry when you notice that:

1. The administration's response to bringing in new programs has been positive, but programs are readily discontinued.

2. The materials are not age and grade appropriate.

3. The program contains few specific guidelines or instructions regarding the everyday details for carrying it out; there is no cadre of implementers in contexts like yours to which you have access.

(continued)

TABLE 9.6 (continued)

4. Program procedures do not include explicit home carry-over activities.
5. The program does not focus sufficiently on issues and concerns relevant to your students.
6. Implementers report that it is difficult to maintain appropriate classroom decorum during program time.
7. A climate of trust among students and teachers regarding the program has been difficult to create.
8. Those carrying out the program express feelings of being "lost" or frustrated.
9. Students do not seem to carry over the behaviors taught in the program into real life.
10. Shortages of funding are used as, or actually serve as, a barrier to program delivery.
11. The level of enthusiasm for the program in the district has declined over time.

that should be encouraged, and those that suggest the long-term future of a program is in jeopardy. There is a combination of historical and current information requested. Each item can be rated along a 4-point scale, with the following anchors: 3 = strongly agree, 2 = agree, 1 = disagree, 0 = strongly disagree. Although extensive norms do not yet exist, the guidelines nevertheless provide a structured and standard way of monitoring priority implementation areas and maintaining a positive balance of forces at work for and against long-term program operation (Elias & Clabby, 1992).

ASSESSING SOCIAL PROBLEM-SOLVING SKILL ACQUISITION

A basic question surrounding any social problem-solving intervention is the extent to which students receiving the program are improving their skills in reacting to and thinking through problems and decisions they face. Some information about this can be derived from the Satisfaction surveys presented earlier. Additional information can be derived from functional assessment, such as examining student performance on thought essays, in small work groups, and in other areas in which their social problem solving skills might be in evidence. Formal assessment tools to measure both readiness and problem-solving and decision-making skills in students also exist, especially at the elementary and middle school levels (Elias, 1993; Elias & Clabby, 1992; Elias, Tobias, & Friedlander, 1994).

Many implementers have found the Checklist of Social Problem-

TABLE 9.7. A Checklist of Students' Social Problem-Solving Strengths across Situations

Child:_____ Date:_____

In what situations is this child able to: *Situations*[a]

A. Self-control skills

   1. Listen carefully and accurately   _____

   2. Remember and follow directions   _____

   3. Concentrate and follow through on tasks   _____

   4. Calm him- or herself down   _____

   5. Carry on a conversation without upsetting or provoking   _____
others

B. Social awareness and group participation skills

   6. Accept praise or approval   _____

   7. Choose praiseworthy and caring friends   _____

   8. Know when help is needed   _____

   9. Ask for help when needed   _____

  10. Work as part of a problem-solving team   _____

C. Social problem-solving and decision-making skills

  11. Recognize signs of feelings in self   _____

  12. Recognize signs of feelings in others   _____

  13. Describe accurately a range of feelings   _____

  14. Put problems into words clearly   _____

  15. State realistic interpersonal goals   _____

  16. Think of several ways to solve a problem or reach a goal   _____

  17. Think of different types of solutions   _____

  18. Do (16) and (17) for different types of problems   _____

  19. Differentiate short- *and* long-term consequences   _____

  20. Look at effects of choices on self and others   _____

  21. Keep positive *and* negative possibilities in mind   _____

  22. Select solutions that can reach goals   _____

  23. Make choices that do not harm self, others   _____

  24. Consider details before carrying out a solution (who,
when, where, with whom, etc.)   _____

  25. Anticipate obstacles to plans   _____

  26. Respond appropriately when plans are thwarted   _____

  27. Try out his or her ideas   _____

  28. Learn from experiences or from seeking input from
adults, friends   _____

  29. Use previous experience to help "next time"   _____

[a]Situations can be recorded by entering the numbers of those situations in which particular skills appear to be demonstrated, using the following codes: 1 = with peers in classroom; 2 = with peers in other situations in school; 3 = with teachers; 4 = with other adults in school; 5 = with parents; 6 = with siblings or other relatives; 7 = with peers outside of school; 8 = when under academic stress or pressure; 9 = when under social or peer-related stress or pressure; 10 = when under family related stress or pressure; 11 = other:_____.

Solving Strengths to be of value in organizing and structuring their observations of students' skills, areas of strength, areas that respond to intervention, and areas in need of further work (see Table 9.7). The Checklist is organized to reflect the use of skills across a variety of interpersonal contexts, including out-of-school venues, because it has been our experience that students often do not exhibit their skills consistently across domains. This inconsistency tends to reflect behavioral norms, reinforcement contingencies, or prompting and cuing patterns that are not linked with, or are perhaps even divergent from, those that will promote generalization of social problem-solving skills. Thus, the checklist is as useful for exploring contexts that need to be made congruent in the social problem-solving messages they give to students as it is useful in pointing out students' individual skills.

With regard to behavioral, attitudinal, or other changes, specific indices can be selected based on expected outcomes. Teacher ratings of prosocial behavior and psychopathology, sociometrics, school records and report card information, self-efficacy and self-concept instruments, as well as student self-report measures of health and of violence, delinquency, substance use, and other antisocial and self-destructive behaviors all have been used in prior studies (Elias & Clabby, 1992; Weissberg & Elias, 1993).

ASSESSING THE IMPACT OF SOCIAL PROBLEM-SOLVING PROGRAMS ON SCHOOL TRANSITIONS

One area of concern is the extent to which prevention programs such as social problem solving assist children in making transitions, especially from school to school. Jason and Associates (1992) have written extensively on the ways in which school transitions impact negatively on children, and have documented the surprising frequency of occurrence of this phenomenon. Bisgay-Dehan (1993) developed a procedure that allows one to track, relatively unobtrusively, those aspects of preparation for school transition that children find most helpful. Her methodology, which was developed in the context of elementary school to middle school transition, allows for a look at the impact of a variety of factors, including those social problem-solving activities to which students have been exposed. The format for the assessment is outlined in Table 9.8.

Such an assessment can be tailored for local circumstances and can be used in conjunction with specific measures of transition adaptation (Elias et al., 1992; Felner & Adan, 1988; Jason & Associates, 1993). The feedback provided can be of immense value to school practitioners at all levels, as well as to parents, in minimizing the destabilizing effects of transitions on many students.

A FINAL WORD: WE HAVE A SPECIAL RESPONSIBILITY

This book is intended to provide school practitioners from diverse disciplines with a brief but practical introduction to a most exciting and relevant area of prosocial and preventive intervention, curriculum, and instruction in the schools. We have attempted to include enough information to allow one to start small, to begin to change one's role, and to gain support and skill in the instructional methods outlined. We and others using social problem solving and decision making have a strong belief that this approach makes a significant contribution to education by making a substantial impact on the way students think and, perhaps most critically, on the ways in which they interact with peers and adults.

Many of the techniques described in this book are complementary to those with which the reader is no doubt familiar. This is not accidental; it reflects our work with practitioners and our goal of developing approaches in a way that allows for creative integration of FIG TESPN and the rest of the social problem-solving framework into the programs already being carried out for the benefit of students. It is tempting to think that what one is doing is so much like what we have described that no change is necessary. This may be the case, but it probably is not. There are key elements—often small things—that matter a great deal when it comes to producing positive outcomes for students. We ask that you engage in careful self-examination, and that you take a leadership role in helping your colleagues do the same. We all are overburdened with the number and nature of our tasks related to children; it therefore behooves us to maximize our impact, which, in the case of social problem solving, may take the form of relatively small but powerful adjustments in how things are done. The force of these changes will be more visible over time than they will be immediately. But, like a relay race, as we run each leg better and faster and hand off the baton to teammates, coworkers, and colleagues more smoothly and in a coordinated manner, we will find ourselves involved in many more winning races.

Why Me?

Having read this, it is natural to look around you and see colleagues that have not read this book, or many other books lately, and perhaps seem not to share your motivation, concern, and dedication to children. As you look around, you also see children with incredible, saddening, often staggering needs. Yet, as we look around, we have come to find that the picture is less bleak than it looks. Many individuals are unsure how to proceed in their work; they are frustrated, burned out, overwhelmed by the challenges they

TABLE 9.8. Survey/Interview of Factors Helpful to School Transition

Part 1: Open-ended questions

1. What did you learn in _____ (previous school) that helped you get ready for _____ (current school)? Try to think of at least five things.

2. What did you learn in _____ (previous school) that was not so helpful in getting you ready for _____ (current school)?

3. What do you think can be done for students who are in _____ (the grade prior to the transition) to help them get ready for _____ school? What ideas do you have? Try to list at least five.

Part 2: Closed-ended questions

[Next to each item, there should be two columns; students are asked to indicate, for the first column, if the item reflects something they learned about in their previous school; in the second column, they are to indicate if they think it will be helpful for current students about to make the transition; the items reflect specific aspects of programming about which one is interested, and would be tailored to the content of one's SPS and other transition-preparation activities; the items below reflect some of the areas of focus in Bisgay-Dehan's (1993) study of a transition to a middle school in a community with nearly a 50% Latino population.]

1. How to make friends

2. How to handle a situation where a stranger is bothering you

3. Finding an adult you can trust to ask for help

4. Keeping calm when you are upset

5. Dangers of using alcohol/smoking cigarettes/taking drugs

6. Handling prejudice (when a person makes fun of you, threatens you, or restricts you because of the color of your skin, your religion, your beliefs, where you come from, or something else about your physical appearance)

7. The traditions and holidays of your cultural/ethnic group

8. Saying "no" when others ask you to do something that you feel you should not do

9. Solving a problem by using problem-solving steps

10. Using an appropriate tone of voice when you speak to someone

11. Sharing your feelings with your friends

12. How to work out a problem with a friend when you have a conflict

---

face, feeling underappreciated, dismayed by the increasing severity and complexity of problems they are facing, and distressed over parents' seeming inability or unwillingness to get as involved as perhaps they should. *But very few have lost the caring that prompted entry into this field* (it certainly was not for financial gain!).

What is needed is leadership, determination, a willingness to step forward, a belief that making small differences with even a fraction of the students in need is worthwhile (indeed, essential), and a framework that is feasible, has been found to be effective, and that can be communicated and shared with others across disciplines. We have attempted to provide the framework; we urge you to provide the rest. Drawing from the words of the ancient sage and scholar Hillel, from the *Pirke Avot* (1:14), each of us must ask, "If I am only for myself, what am I? If not now, when?"

♦♦♦

Think Now for Later

♦

KEEPING YOUR BODY IN SHAPE

Every day, each of us makes many decisions that affect our health. We choose what to eat, when to eat, and how much to eat. We decide when and how to keep our bodies clean. We think about the air we breathe and try to keep it clean. And we all know what happens if we are not careful with our decisions. Just think about a time you have eaten too much, or you have eaten too late at night. What a lousy feeling in your stomach and your whole body! And when you haven't kept clean, you probably remember how your hair might have felt itchy and greasy. You didn't look your best and maybe your skin even got worse. Everybody knows how awful it is when the air isn't clean. Just think about how horrible it is when you drive past the oil refineries on the turnpike or when you come into a room filled with cigarette smoke or, even worse, cigar smoke. Being healthy and living in a healthy world involves, as we said in the beginning, decisions and choices. What exactly is a "decision"? What exactly is a "choice"? Go look up these words in a dictionary and write the meanings either in the spaces below or on an answer sheet.

Decision: _____

_____

_____

_____

Choice: _____

_____

_____

_____

As you found out, both decisions and choices involve *thinking* about what you want to have happen and different ways of getting things to happen. To make a good, healthy decision, you have to know what your goals are. Bad decisions—decisions that will make you less healthy, make you less alert, and make your body less able to do what you want it to—are usually made because people are not sure what their goals are. They aren't thinking about *the future.* They aren't *thinking now for later*

Bad decisions are decisions that end up harming your body or your mind. They make you less healthy, not more healthy. Smoking, taking drugs, abusing alcohol—these are not things that "everybody" does. These things happen to people who make *bad decisions*, who don't think now for later.

Nobody will ever tell you it's smart to smoke, take drugs, or abuse alcohol. Nobody does it because it's smart.

Nobody ever smokes, takes drugs, or drinks to impress their parents or teachers. Nobody does it because they think adults who care about them will be proud of them.

So why do people smoke or use smokeless tobacco or take drugs or abuse alcohol? Because they have made *bad decisions.* They didn't *think now for later.* Most of them will never admit it, even if you ask them. Many people are afraid to say, "I made a bad decision." It doesn't mean they are bad people. But it does mean they made a bad decision and until they stop what they are doing and make new choices, they are harming their bodies or their minds or *both.*

And people who make bad decisions about their health are *ashamed.* So what do they do? Right! *They try to make their bad decision sound good!* And they try to get others to do what they do. Because if you drink or smoke too, then you won't be able to say anything. Deep down, you'll feel ashamed, you body will feel different, and your mind will not be the same.

People don't like to admit this kind of stuff, so, instead, they make it all sound cool and nice and wonderful. But if you *think now for later*, you will decide how this will affect your body and your mind—your *only* body and your *only* mind.

When you *think now for later*, you ask yourself, "Is this going to hurt me, or make me weak or sick or less alert?" If the answer is yes, you should decide not to do it. And if you're not sure, do you think it is a good decision to try it and see? Or would a better decision be to learn more, to find out more from someone who thinks now for later. And who is doing it? Remember, if you *think now for later*, you will make better decisions and better choices and be a healthier, more alert person!

WHAT CAN HAPPEN IF YOU DON'T AND IF YOU DO

We stay healthy because we make decisions and choices that do not harm our bodies or our minds. Sure, it's easy to skip a shower or not bother to brush our teeth. It may seem easy to say "yes" when someone offers you a cigarette or a beer. But if we *think now for later*, we will make better, healthier decisions. After all, who loses if we have skin problems, spend our afternoons in a dentist's chair, or ruin our lungs—we do!

Let's take a look at some children your age who are in the middle of making important decisions and choices about their health. As you read, ask yourself how you might feel if you were Charlie or Warren. Which of them is *thinking now for later?*

Going Down the Tobacco Road . . . or the Healthy Road?

Warren and Charlie were watching television at Charlie's house. They were getting ready for Monday at West End Middle School. They had watched for most of the day, because it was too rainy to do much outside. Warren was watching a commercial for smokeless tobacco. "Boy," he said to himself, "that guy is really cool. And it looks so easy. You just stick it in your lip, and, wow, you'd probably feel great. I'd like to look just like that guy on TV. Even on television, some of those cool cops and other guys have been doing smokeless tobacco instead of smoking. Maybe I'll stop smoking and get some of that tobacco stuff." Charlie was watching the same thing, but had some different thoughts. "Wow," he said to himself, "that guy looks pretty cool. And it sure sounds easy to do. But I wonder what that stuff can do to your lip and mouth? I read somewhere that some of the stuff in tobacco is the same stuff that makes cigarettes give you cancer. Can you imagine having cancer in your mouth? All the sores and everything. . . . How could you eat pizza and ice cream and donuts? Smoking may hurt you, but that smokeless tobacco stuff seems just as dumb to me. There are smarter ways to be cool."

At school the next day, Warren saw Charlie. "Hey, Charlie, you wanna try some of this smokeless stuff? I saw it on TV and it looked really great." "No thanks, Warren. I don't want sores and junk in my mouth." "But didn't you see that guy on TV? He said it was easy." "Yeah, but he didn't say what would happen after a while. I bet he just uses it during commercials."

Warren and Charlie watched the same commercial but thought about it very differently. Charlie is thinking about his health—he's *thinking now for later*. What is Warren thinking about? His goal is to be cool, to feel "great," or to do what's "easy." It's not bad to be "cool," but when the choice is between being cool or being healthy, it's important to *think now for later*. There are other ways to be cool or feel great without cigarettes or smokeless tobacco. Charlie chooses the road to health, and keeps his mouth from getting sores, and maybe cancer, later on.

Let's meet two girls your age who are trying to do their schoolwork but have different ideas about what to do when the work gets hard, or just boring. As you read, think about Janet, Carol, and Katie and who you know in your school who is like each of them.

Pills for Thrills . . . or Poison for Your Body?

Carol was over at Janet's house. They were studying together for a test in social studies, and then they were going to work on a book report for english. They had been working about an hour or so, when Carol started to get restless. "This is boring," Carol said. "I can't stand this." Carol got up and went into the bathroom. She came out after a couple of minutes and showed a bottle of pills to Janet. "Do you want one?" "What's that?" "Oh, these are some pills I take when I get bored or down or sad. I got them from Katie, you know that ninth grader who hangs around when we get out of middle school." "Her? Boy, I wouldn't even trust her to give me a pretzel. Did you ever take a good look at her?" Carol stopped to think. "No, I never have," she said. "Well, you should. She's all skinny and wasted and she looks like she hasn't slept in a month. What a wreck!"

All of a sudden, they heard a key in the door—Janet's parents were back. Carol rushed to put the pills in her book bag. Janet was really surprised at the panic-stricken look on Carol's face. "Carol, you looked so scared," "Yeah, well, these pills are illegal—you can get in trouble if you get caught with them." "Why?" asked Janet. "I don't know," Carol said. "Maybe you should have a prescription or something." Janet said, "Well, then how do you know what's in it, or where it comes from, or how much to take?" Carol was getting annoyed. She said, "Katie told me it was okay. Besides, I get to go to her house and see her friends and listen to her stereo tapes and use her headphones. You ought to come!"

Janet thought for a minute. Katie seemed like a loser. And those pills could be really dangerous. Real medicine is made carefully, in clean places, and with doses that a doctor says are right for you. These pills are, well, very risky . . . *too* risky, thought Janet. But Katie had older friends, a great stereo, and some parties that were really wild. It might be exciting to be her friend . . .

Janet finally answered, "No, I don't think so. It wouldn't be worth hurting myself, maybe really badly, just to be Katie's friend or go to her house. She's no friend if she tries to get you to take pills."

Janet faced some hard choices. What were all the reasons for her to try the pills? When Carol's parents came home, what happened? Was Carol proud of what she did or was she ashamed and scared? Would you choose seeing older kids and using a good stereo if it meant losing your health? Was Carol *thinking now for later*?

When Carol said to Janet, "Do you want one?" she was really asking, "DO YOU WANT TO POISON YOUR BODY?" And we know this is true, because we know about Katie. Janet noticed how Katie looked—awful. Carol never let herself see what pills had done to Katie—and what they would do to her or anyone who tries them. Carol didn't *think now for later*. Sure, there might be some fun hours with Katie and her cool friends, but the clock would strike midnight, and the magic spell would be broken. Carol would have to come back to reality. And if she became addicted to pills— the road back to health would be harder. Janet would always remember:

> When anyone asks you to try pills, drugs, or alcohol . . .
> They are really asking, "DO YOU WANT TO POISON YOUR BODY?"
> If you say "Yes" to be cool, you may end up as a fool.
> If you say "Yes" to feel great, you will end up with a sad fate.

Finally, we are going to meet Robert and Connie. Both have health problems that require visits to the doctor pretty often. They also have to take medication and do special treatments. This is true for many children and teens, such as those with asthma, allergies, diabetes, and, in a similar way, for other youngsters with problems that are mostly physical. Having to take care of yourself so carefully can be a pain. But it s also a *choice*, a *decision about your health*. Let's see what Robert and Connie are feeling and thinking, as they get ready for yet another visit to the doctor.

Not Following Doctor's Orders: Putting One Over . . . or Putting Yourself Under?

When Robert walked into the doctor's office, he was surprised to see Connie in the waiting room. Robert and Connie were both classmates at Hagalil Middle School. They were both at the doctor's for check-ups. Robert had asthma and Connie had allergies. They both had to take medications and do certain breathing exercises. And they both didn't like to do these things.

"Hi, Connie. Isn't this a real drag? My parents schlep me here every two weeks. I really hate it!" "So do I. Every morning they bother me to take the medicine, take the medicine, take the medicine. Sometimes I just pretend to take it, and then I throw it out." Robert looked surprised. "You do? Why?" Connie said, "They hassle me so much that I've got to do *something*. So, I show them. I put those tablets in my cheek and spit them out in the bathroom."

Robert thought about what Connie said. He also hated the medicine, the doctor's visits, and the breathing machine. But he never thought about doing what Connie did. Sure, he got upset at his parents for always reminding him. But what if he didn't take the medicine? He'd probably feel the same for a little while, but after a few days—big trouble! It didn't make any sense to hurt himself just because he was angry at his parents.

"Connie, I don't understand why you pretend with the pills. It just hurts you!" "But I've *got* to do *something*. I didn't ask to be sick, and at least I can show my parents that I have some choices that are mine." "Connie, that doesn't make any sense. If you want to show you can do stuff, show it in some other way, maybe with your writing or your music or something else. You're good at *those* things. It just seems weird to take a chance on making yourself sicker when you're upset about being sick! You'll end up with more medicines and treatments!"

Now it was Connie's turn to do a little thinking.

If you were Connie, what would you be thinking? Perhaps you'd say to yourself, "I definitely have a problem. I hate these medicines. I hate being sick. And I hate everybody telling me what to do and how to do it. Well, I *do* have allergies and I can't wish them away. And when I get an attack, wow, it sure is painful. Once they even thought I'd die! What do I want most that I *can* have?"

"Connie's answer would probably be to show her parents, and others, that there is a lot she can do. But if she doesn't take her medicine, how would that help? If her parents found out—and they probably would, when she had an attack—they might ground her. And they *certainly* wouldn't trust her. If you were Connie, it would probably be a good idea to *think now for later*. Do what has to be done to *stay healthy*. Your parents will trust you and you will feel as well as *you* can feel. Then, you can think of different ways of showing what you can do, or how you feel. Robert had two good suggestions for Connie: writing or music. It's natural to get angry at doctors or your parents or medicine or treatments. But if you *think now for later*, you'll remember how things would be *without* medicine and treatment. By putting one over on the doctors, you may really be putting yourself under.

Wrapping It Up: It's Your Body and Your Mind

There are many important decisions and choices that we have to make about our health. Sometimes, our friends or people we know will make suggestions that may seem good at the time. But if we *think now for later*, we might realize that we can poison our body or poison our mind if we follow their ideas. It can be hard to say "No," to resist these ideas. What will your friends think? Will they reject you or tease you? Charlie, Janet, and Robert thought and made decisions that will be good for their health. It wasn't easy, but they told their friends they wouldn't follow along, that it is more important to be healthy than to be "cool" or try to show adults that you can put one over on them. You have one body and one mind— if you choose *now* to keep them both healthy, you'll have them in good working condition for lots of fun things *later*.

APPENDIX B

♦♦♦

Listing of Resources

♦

STUDENT CONFLICT MANAGER

The Student Conflict Manager/Personal Problem Solving Guide has been developed by Psychological Enterprises, 160 Hanover Avenue, Suite 103, Cedar Knolls, NJ 07927. For information about ordering, volume discounts, or site licenses, please call 201-829-6806. There also is a fax line available at 201-829-6802.

TALKING WITH TJ

To order *Talking with TJ*, call 1-800-ORDER TJ or write to Talking with TJ Orders, 1002 N. 42nd Street, Omaha, NE 68131-9834. The approximate cost of each three-video series, including curriculum materials and leaders' guide, is $25.

MATERIALS FOR EDUCATORS

Social decision making and life skills development: Guidelines for middle school educators (M. J. Elias, Ed., 1993). Aspen Publishers, 200 Orchard Ridge Drive, Gaithersburg, MD 20878; 1-800-638-8437.

Building social problem solving skills: Guidelines from a school-based program (M. J. Elias & J. F. Clabby, 1992). Jossey-Bass Publishers, 350 Sansome Street, San Francisco, CA 94104; 1-800-956-7739.

Social decision making skills: A curriculum guide for the elementary grades (M. J. Elias & J. F. Clabby, 1989). Aspen Publishers, 200 Orchard Ridge Drive, Gaithersburg, MD 20878; 1-800-638-8437.

MATERIALS FOR PARENTS

Teach your child decision making (J. F. Clabby & M. J. Elias, 1986). Psychological Enterprises, 160 Hanover Avenue, Suite 103, Cedar Knolls, NJ 07927; 1-201-829-6806.

References

♦

Agency for Instructional Technology. (1994). *Catalog of instructional materials.* Bloomington, IN: Author.

Ager, C., & Cole, C. (1991). A review of cognitive behavioral interventions for children and adolescents with behavioral disorders. *Behavioral Disorders, 16,* 275–287.

Alexander, F., & Crabtree, C. (1988). California's new history -social science curriculum promises richness and depth. *Educational Leadership, 46,* 10–13.

Armstrong, T. (1994). *Multiple intelligences in the classroom.* Alexandria, VA: Association for Supervision and Curriculum Development.

Asarnow, J., Carlson, G., & Guthrie, D. (1987). Coping strategies, self-perceptions, hopelessness, and perceived family environments in depressed and suicidal children. *Journal of Consulting and Clinical Psychology, 55,* 361–336.

Baron, J., & Brown, R. (Eds.). (1991). *Teaching decision making to adolescents.* Hillsdale, NJ: Erlbaum.

Basch. C. E. (1983). Research on disseminating and implementing health education programs in the schools. *Journal of School Health, 54,* 57–66.

Battistich, V.A ., Elias, M. J., & Branden-Muller, L. R. (1992). Two school-based approaches to promoting children's social competence. In G. W. Albee, L. A. Bond, & T. V. Cook-Monsey (Eds.), *Improving children's lives: Global perspectives on prevention* (pp. 217–234). Newbury Park, CA: Sage.

Benard, B., Fafoglia, G., & Perone, J. (1987, February). Knowing what to do and not to do— reinvigorates drug education. *Association for Supervision and Curriculum Development Curriculum Update,* pp. 1–12.

Bhaerman, R. D. & Kopp, K. A. (1988). *The school's choice: Guidelines for drop-out prevention at the middle and junior high school* (Drop-out Prevention Series). Columbus, OH: National Center for Research in Vocational Education. (ERIC-Document Reproduction Service No. ED 298 324)

Bisgay-Dehan, K. (1993). *The middle school transition: An exploratory study of the personal and environmental characteristics associated with students' adaptation.* Unpublished doctoral dissertation, Graduate School of Applied and Professional Psychology, Rutgers University. New Brunswick, NJ.

Botvin, G. J. (1985). The Life Skills Training Program as a health promotion strategy: Theoretical issues and empirical findings. In J. Zins, D. Wagner, & C. Maher (Eds.), *Health promotion in the schools* (pp. 9–23). New York: Haworth Press.

Braaten, S., Kauffman, J. M., Braaten, B., Posgrove, L., & Nelson, C. M. (1988). The Regular Education Initiative: Potent medicine for behavioral disorders. *Exceptional Children, 55,* 21–27.

Bransford, J., Sherwood, R., Vye, N., & Rieser, J. (1986). Teaching thinking and problem solving: Research foundations. *American Psychologist, 41,* 1078–1089.

Braswell, L. (1993). Cognitive-behavioral groups for children manifesting ADHD and other disruptive behavior disorders. In J. Zins & M. Elias (Eds.), *Promoting student success through group interventions* (pp. 91–116). New York: Haworth Press.

Braswell, L., & Bloomquist, M. L. (1991). *Cognitive-behavioral therapy with ADHD children: Child, family, and school interventions.* New York: Guilford Press.

Brendtro, L., Brokenleg, M., & Van Bockern, S. (1991). The circle of courage. *Beyond Behavior, 2*(1), 5–12.

Bronfenbrenner, U. (1979). Contexts of child rearing: Problems and prospects. *American Psychologist, 34,* 844–850.

Bruene-Butler, L., Schuyler, T., & Clabby, J. F. (1993). *Manual for training of certified trainers in the Social Decision Making and Problem Solving Program.* Piscataway, NJ: UMDNJ-CMHC SPS Unit.

Burch, P. (1992). *The drop-out problem in New Jersey's big urban schools: Educational inequality and governmental inaction.* New Brunswick, NJ: Rutgers University.

Carnine, D. (1994). Introduction to the mini-series: Educational tools for diverse learners. *School Psychology Review, 23,* 341–350.

Cartledge, G., & Milburn, J. (Eds.). (1984). *Teaching social skills to children* (rev. ed.). New York: Pergamon Press.

Centers for Disease Control (1988). *Guidelines for effective school health education to prevent the spread of AIDS* (DHHS Publication No. CDC 88–8017). Atlanta: Author.

Clabby, J. F., & Elias, M. J. (1986). *Teach your child decision making.* Available from Psychological Enterprises Incorporated, 160 Hanover Avenue, Suite 103, Cedar Knolls, NJ 07927

Copple, C., Sigel, I., & Saunders, R. (1979). *Educating the young thinker.* New York: Van Nostrand.

Cornell Cooperative Extension (1989). *Nutrition education curriculum.* Ithaca, NY: Author.

Crabbe, A. (1989). The future problem solving program. *Educational Leadership, 46,* 27–29.

DeBock, A., & Paul, C. (1989). One district's commitment to global education. *Educational Leadership, 44,* 46–49.

Educational Development Corporation. (1994). *Teenage health teaching modules.* Boston: Author.

Elias, M. J. (1982). Using programs for emotionally disturbed children in mainstreamed or special class settings. In B. Baskin & R. Harris (Eds.), *The mainstreamed library: Issues, ideas, innovations* (pp. 178–186). Chicago: American Library Association.

Elias, M. J. (1983). Improving coping skills of emotionally disturbed boys through television-based social problem solving. *American Journal of Orthopsychiatry, 53,* 61–72.

Elias, M. J. (1989). Schools as a source of stress to children: An analysis of causal and ameliorative influences. *Journal of School Psychology, 27,* 393–407.

Elias, M. J. (1990). The role of affect and social relationships in health behavior and school health curriculum and instruction. *Journal of School Health, 60,* 157–163.

Elias, M. J. (Ed.). (1993). *Social decision making and life skills development: Guidelines for middle school educators.* Gaithersburg, MD: Aspen.

Elias, M. J., & Clabby, J.F. (1989). *Social decision making skills: A curriculum guide for the elementary grades.* Gaithersburg, MD: Aspen.

Elias, M. J., & Clabby, J.F. (1992). *Building social problem solving skills: Guidelines from a school-based program.* San Francisco: Jossey-Bass.

Elias, M. J., Gager, P., & Hancock, M. (1993). *Preventive and social competence programs in use in New Jersey public schools: Findings from a statewide survey: An executive summary of a report from the School Intervention Implementation Study.* New Brunswick, NJ: Rutgers University, Department of Psychology.

Elias, M. J., Gager, P., & Hancock, M. (1994). *Conditions for implementing prevention programs in high-risk environments: Application of the resiliency paradigm.* Manuscript under review.

Elias, M. J., Gara, M. A., Schuyler, T. F., Branden-Muller, L. R., & Sayette, M. A. (1991). The promotion of social competence: Longitudinal study of a preventive school-based program. *American Journal of Orthopsychiatry, 61,* 409–417.

Elias, M. J., Gara, M., & Ubriaco, M. (1985). Sources of stress and support in children's transition to middle school: An empirical analysis. *Journal of Clinical Child Psychology, 14,* 112–118.

Elias, M. J., Gara, M., Ubriaco, M., Rothbaum, P. A., Clabby, J. F., & Schuyler, T. (1986). The impact of a preventive social problem solving intervention on children's coping with middle school stressors. *American Journal of Community Psychology, 14,* 259–275.

Elias, M. J., Hancock, M., Gager, P., & Chung, H. (1993). Promoting a multicultural perspective in students. In M. J. Elias (Ed.), *Social decision making and life skills development: Guidelines for middle school educators* (pp. 251–260). Gaithersburg, MD: Aspen.

Elias, M. J., Tobias, S.E., & Friedlander, B.S. (1994). Enhancing skills for everyday problem solving, decision making, and conflict resolution in special needs students with the support of computer-based technology. *Special Services in the Schools, 8,* 33–52.

Elias, M. J., Ubriaco, M., Reese, A., Gara, M., Rothbaum, P., & Haviland, M. (1992). A measure of adaptation to problematic academic and interpersonal tasks of middle school. *Journal of School Psychology, 30,* 41–57.

Elias, M. J., & Weissberg, R. P. (1990). School-based social competence promotion as a primary prevention strategy: A tale of two projects. In R. Lorion (Ed.), *Protecting the children: Strategies for optimizing human development* (pp. 177–200). New York: Haworth.

Elias, M. J., Weissberg, R., Dodge, K., Hawkins, J. D., Kendall, P., Jason, L., Perry,

C., Rotheram-Borus, M. J., & Zins, J. E. (1994). The school-based promotion of social competence: Theory, research, and practice. In R. Haggerty, L. Sherrod, N. Garmezy, & M. Rutter, (Eds.), *Stress, risk, and resilience, in children and adolescents* (pp. 268–316). New York: Cambridge University Press.

Epstein, T., Elias, M. J., & Lefkowitz, D. (1995). *"Talking with TJ": A formative evaluation of the application of a video-based, multicultural social competence promotion and violence prevention intervention to after school day care settings.* Manuscript under review.

Felner, R. D., & Adan, A. (1988). The school transitional environmental project: An ecological intervention and evaluation. In R. H. Price, E. L. Cowen, R. P. Lorion, & J. Ramos-McKay (Eds.), *Fourteen ounces of prevention: A casebook for practitioners* (pp. 111–122). Washington, DC: American Psychological Association.

Flaherty, E., Mracek, J., Olsen, R., & Wilcove, G. (1983). Preventing adolescent pregnancy: An interpersonal problem solving approach. *Prevention in Human Services, 2,* 49–64.

Fox, C. L. (1989). Peer acceptance of learning disabled children in the regular classroom. *Exceptional Children, 56,* 50–59.

Freedman, B., Donahoe, C., Rosenthal, L., Schlundt, D., & McFall, R. (1978). A social-behavioral analysis of skill deficits in delinquent and nondelinquent boys. *Journal of Consulting and Clinical Psychology, 46,* 1448–1462.

Friedlander, B. (1993). Incorporating computer technologies into social decision making: Applications to problem behavior. In M. J. Elias (Ed.), *Social decision making and life skills development: Guideline for middle school educators* (pp. 315–318). Gaithersburg, MD: Aspen.

Fuchs, D., & Fuchs, L. S. (1994). Inclusive schools movement and the radicalization of special education reform. *Exceptional Children, 60,* 294–309.

Fullan, M. (1993). *Change forces: Probing the depths of educational reform.* Bristol, PA: Falmer Press.

Gardner, H. (1993). *The multiple intelligences: The theory in practice.* New York: Basic Books.

Gartner, A., & Lipsky, D. K. (1987). Beyond special education: Toward a quality system for all students. *Harvard Educational Review, 57,* 367–395.

Gibbs, J. T. (1989). Black American adolescents. In J. T. Gibbs & L. N. Huang (Eds.), *Children of color: Psychological intervention with minority youth* (pp. 179–223). San Francisco: Jossey-Bass.

Goldstein, A., Sprafkin, R. Gershaw, N. & Klein, P. (1980). *Skillstreaming the adolescent.* Champaign, IL: Research Press.

Gopin, M., Levine, M., & Schwartz, S. (1994). *Jewish civics: A tikkun olam/world repair manual.* New York: Coalition for the Advancement of Jewish Education.

Gordon, S., & Asher, M. (1994). *Meeting the ADD challenge: A practical guide for teachers.* Champaign, IL: Research Press.

Grady, K., Kline, M., Belanoff, L., & Snow, D. (1993). Guiding your child's decisions: Programs for parents. In M. J. Elias (Ed.), *Social decision making and life skills development: Guidelines for middle school educators* (pp. 207–238). Gaithersburg, MD: Aspen.

Gresham. F. M. (1982). Misguided mainstreaming: The case for social skills training with handicapped children. *Exceptional Children, 48*, 422–433.

Gresham. F. M. (1984). Social skills and self efficacy for exceptional children. *Exceptional Children, 51*, 253–261.

Gresham, F. M., & Elliott, S.N. (1993). Social skills intervention guide: Systematic approaches to social skills training. In J. E. Zins & M. J. Elias (Eds.), *Promoting student success through group interventions* (pp. 137–158). New York: Haworth Press.

Haboush, K., & Elias, M. J. (1993). The social decision making approach to social studies, citizenship, and critical thinking. In M. J. Elias, *Social decision making and life skills development: Guidelines for middle school educators* (pp. 79–104). Gaithersburg, MD: Aspen.

Hallmark Corporate Foundation. (1994). *Talking with TJ: A new educational resource to teach teamwork, cooperation, and conflict resolution.* Omaha, NE: Author.

Halper, A., Klepp, R., Murray, D., Perry, C., & Smyth, M. (1986). *The Minnesota Smoking Prevention Program.* Minneapolis: University of Minnesota School of Public Health.

Hawkins, J., Doueck, H., & Lishner, D. (1988). Changing teaching practices in mainstream classrooms to improve bonding and behavior of low achievers. *American Educational Research Journal, 25*, 31–50.

Hechinger, F. M. (1992). *Fateful choices: Healthy youth for the 21st century.* New York: Carnegie Council on Adolescent Development/Carnegie Corporation of New York.

Hett, C., & Clabby, J. (1993). Curriculum procedures for the self-contained special education classroom. In M. J. Elias (Ed.), *Social decision making and life skills development: Guidelines for middle school educators* (pp. 175–206). Gaithersburg, MD: Aspen.

Hett, C., & Krikorian, L. (1993). Fostering communication through school and home newsletters. In M. J. Elias, *Social decision making and life skills development: Guidelines for middle school educators* (pp. 261–272). Gaithersburg, MD: Aspen.

Huberman, M., & Miles, M. (1984). *Innovation up close: How school improvement works.* New York: Plenum.

Irwin, C. D., Jr. (Ed.). (1987). *Adolescent social behavior and health: New directions for child development* (No. 37). San Francisco: Jossey-Bass.

Isaac, K. (1992). *Civics for democracy: A journey for teachers and students.* Washington, DC: Center for the Study of Responsive Law.

Jason, L., Weine, A., Johnson, J., Warren-Sohlberg, L., Filippelli, L., Turner, E., & Lardon, C. (1992). *Helping transfer students: Strategies for educational and social readjustment.* San Francisco: Jossey-Bass.

Jessor, R. (1991). Risk behavior in adolescence: A psychosocial framework for understanding and action. *Journal of Adolescent Health, 12*, 597–605.

Johnson, D., & Johnson, R. (1990). Social skills for successful group work. *Educational Leadership, 47*(4), 29–33.

Johnson, D., Johnson, R., Dudley, B., & Burnett, R. (1992). Teaching students to be peer mediators. *Educational Leadership, 50*, 10–13.

Johnson, R., & Bruene-Butler, L. (1993). Promoting social decision making skills of middle school students: A school/community/environmental service project.

In M. J. Elias (Ed.), *Social decision making and life skills development: Guidelines for middle school educators* (pp. 241–250). Gaithersburg, MD: Aspen.

Jones, V. (1991). Responding to students' behavior problems. *Beyond Behavior, 2*(1), 17–21.

Jordan, I. K. (1993). A matter of access: Technology for deaf and hard-of-hearing people. *Technos, 2*(2), 26–28.

Kazdin, A., & Associates. (1987). Problem solving skills training and relationship therapy in the treatment of antisocial child behavior. *Journal of Consulting and Clinical Psychology, 55,* 76–85.

Kendall, P.C. (1988). *Stop and think workbook.* (Available from the author, 238 Meeting House Lane, Merion Station, PA 19066.)

King, D. (1986, June). Broad-based support pushes health education beyond what the coach does between sessions. *Association for Supervision and Curriculum Development Curriculum Update,* pp. 1–8.

Kniep, W. (1986). Defining a global education by its content. *Social Education, 50,* 437–445.

Kolbe, L. (1985). Why school health education? An empirical point of view. *Health Education, 16,* 116–120.

Lawrence, S. (1989). National standards and local portraits. *Teachers College Record, 91,* 14–17.

Levine, D. (1988). Teaching thinking to at-risk students: Generalizations and speculation. In B. Presseisen (Ed.), *At-risk students and thinking: Perspectives from research* (pp. 117–137). Washington, DC: National Education Association/Research for Better Schools.

Lickona, T. (1991). *Educating for character: How our schools can teach respect and responsibility.* New York: Bantam Books.

Lipman, M. (1988). Critical thinking: What can it be? *Educational Leadership, 46,* 38–43.

London, P. (1987). Character education and clinical intervention: A paradigm shift for U.S. schools. *Phi Delta Kappan, 68,* 667–673.

Mahood, W. (1981, January). Born losers: School drop-outs and pushouts. *NASSP Bulletin, 65*(441), 54–57.

McCarthy, B. (1990). Using the 4MAT system to bring learning styles to schools. *Educational Leadership, 47,* 31–37.

McIntosh, R., Vaughn, S., & Zaragoza, N. (1991). A review of social interventions for students with learning disabilities. *Journal of Learning Disabilities, 24,* 451–458.

Meier, D. (1989). Comment on the National Standards for American Education symposium. *Teachers College Record, 91,* 25–27.

Miller, M. G., Midgett, J., & Wicks, M. L. (1992). Student and teacher perceptions related to behavior change after skillstreaming training. *Behavioral Disorders, 17,* 291–295.

Mirman, J., Swartz, R., & Barell, J. (1988). Strategies to help teachers empower at-risk students. In B. Presseisen (Ed.), *At-risk students and thinking: Perspectives from research* (pp. 138–156). Washington, DC: National Education Association/Research for Better Schools.

Naftel, M., & Elias, M. J. (1995). Building problem solving and decision making skills through literature analysis. *Middle School Journal, 26*(4), 7–11.

National Center for Health Education. (1985). *Growing healthy: Comprehensive school health education program guide.* New York: American Lung Association.

National Education Goals Panel. (1994). *The National Education Goals Panel Report: Building a nation of learners, 1994.* Washington, DC: U.S. Government Printing Office.

National Professional School Health Organizations. (1984). Comprehensive school health education. *Journal of School Health, 54,* 312–315

Natriello, G., Pallas, A., & McDill, E. (1986). Taking stock: Renewing our research agenda on the causes and consequences of dropping out. *Teachers College Record, 87*(3), 430–440.

Natriello, G., Pallas, A., McDill, E., McPartland, J., & Royster, D. (1988). *An examination of the assumptions and evidence for alternative drop-out prevention programs in high school* (Report No. 365). Baltimore, MD: Johns Hopkins University, Center for Research on Elementary and Middle Schools. (ERIC Document Reproduction Service No. ED 299 374)

Nigro, L. (1995). *The Social Problem Solving Lab: Pre-referral intervention to enhance elementary students' critical thinking skills.* Unpublished doctoral dissertation, Graduate School of Applied and Professional Psychology, Rutgers University, New Brunswick, NJ.

Oregon Research Institute. (1986). *Project PATH: Programs to advance teen health.* Eugene, OR: Oregon Research Institute.

Orr, M. (1987). *Keeping students in school: A guide to effective drop-out prevention programs and services.* San Francisco: Jossey-Bass.

Palincsar, A., & Brown, A. (1985). Reciprocal teaching: Activities to promote "reading with your mind." In T. Harris & E. Cooper (Eds.), *Reading, thinking, and concept development: Strategies for the classroom* (pp. 147–160). New York: College Entrance Examination Board.

Panel on High Risk Youth of the National Research Council (1993). *Losing generations: Adolescents in high-risk settings.* Washington, DC: National Academy Press.

Papke, M., & Elias, M. J. (1993). Tools for monitoring and evaluating middle school programs. In M. J. Elias (Ed.), *Social decision making and life skills development: Guidelines for middle school educators* (pp. 273–300). Gaithersburg, MD: Aspen.

Patterson, G. (1975). *Families: Applications of social learning theory to family life.* Champaign, IL: Research Press.

Perkins, D. (1986). Thinking frames. *Educational Leadership, 43,* 4–11.

Psychological Enterprises Incorporated. (1993). *The Student Conflict Manager/Personal Problem Solving Guide.* Cedar Knolls, NJ: Author.

Purdy, C. & Tritsch, L. (1985). Why school health education? The practical point of view. *Health Education, 16,* 110–112.

Quigley, C., & Bahmueller, C. (1991). *CIVITAS: A framework for civic education.* Calabasas, CA: Center for Civic Education.

Raven, J. (1987). Values, diversity, and cognitive development. *Teachers College Record, 89,* 21–38.

Rosado, J. W., Jr. (1986). Toward an interfacing of Hispanic cultural variables with school psychology service delivery systems. *Professional Psychology: Research and Practice, 17,* 191–199.

Rubinstein, H. (1993). How television can encourage critical thinking: Using video power to teach social decision making skills. In M. J. Elias, *Social decision making and life skills development: Guidelines for middle school educators* (pp. 139–174). Gaithersburg, MD: Aspen.

Rutter, M. (1987). Psychosocial resilience and protective mechanisms. *American Journal of Orthopsychiatry, 57,* 316–331.

Salomon, G. (1979). *The interaction of media, cognition and learning.* San Francisco: Jossey-Bass.

Sarason, S. B. (1982). *The culture of the school and the problem of change* (2nd ed.). Boston: Allyn & Bacon.

Sarason, S. B. (1990). Forging the classroom's "Constitutions." *Education Week, 10*(8), 27, 36.

Schloss, P. J. (1992). Mainstreaming revisited. *Elementary School Journal, 92,* 233–244.

Schrag, J., & Burnette, J. (1994). Inclusive schools. *Teaching Exceptional Children, 26,* 64–68.

Scruggs, T., Mastropieri, M., & Sullivan, G. S. (1994). Promoting relational thinking: Elaborative interrogation for students with mild disabilities. *Exceptional Children, 60,* 450–457.

Shinn, M., & McConnell, S. (1994). Improving general education instruction: Relevance to school psychologists. *School Psychology Review, 23,* 351–371.

Shure, M. (1994). *I Can Problem Solve (ICPS): An interpersonal cognitive problem-solving program for children.* Champaign, IL: Research Press.

Slavin, R. (1990). Research on cooperative learning: Consensus and controversy. *Educational Leadership, 47*(4), 52–55.

Small, R., & Schinke, S. (1983). Teaching competence in residential group care: Cognitive problem solving and interpersonal training with emotionally disturbed adolescents. *Journal of Social Services Research, 7,* 1–16.

Spivack, G., Platt, J. J. Jr., & Shure, M. (1976). *The problem solving approach to adjustment.* San Francisco: Jossey-Bass.

Stainback, S., Stainback, W., East, K., & Sapon-Shevin, M. (1994). A commentary on inclusion and the development of a positive self-identity by people with disabilities. *Exceptional Children, 60,* 486–490.

Sternberg, R., & Wagner, R. (Eds.). (1986). *Practical intelligence: Nature and organization of competence in the everyday world.* Cambridge, United Kingdom: Cambridge University Press.

Tobias, S. E. (1992). *FIG TESPN goes to middle school: An intervention guide.* Cedar Knolls, NJ: Psychological Enterprises.

Using videotape technology to build special education students' social skills [Special issue]. *Teaching Exceptional Children, 27*(3), 4–22.

Valentine, M. R. (1987). *How to deal with discipline problems in the schools: A practical guide for educators.* Dubuque, IA: Kendall/Hunt.

Wales, C., Nardi, A., & Stager, R. (1986). Decision making: A new paradigm for education. *Educational Leadership, 2,* 37–42.

Weissberg, R. P. (1985). Designing effective social problem solving problems for the classroom. In B. Schneider, R. H. Rubin, & J. Ledingham (Eds.), *Peer relationships and social skills in childhood: Vol. 2. Issues in assessment and training* (pp. 225–242). New York: Springer-Verlag.

Weissberg, R. P., & Elias, M. J. (1993). Enhancing young people's social competence and health behavior: An important challenge for educators, scientists, policymakers, and funders. *Applied & Preventive Psychology, 2,* 179–190.

Weissberg, R., Jackson, A., & Shriver, T. (1993). Promoting positive social development and health practices in young urban adolescents. In M. J. Elias (Ed.), *Social decision making and life skills development: Guidelines for middle school educators* (pp. 45–78). Gaithersburg, MD: Aspen.

Wells, S. (1990). *At-risk youth: Identification, programs and Recommendations.* Englewood, CO: Teacher Idea Press.

Willis, S. (1993). Schools test new ways to resolve conflict. *ASCD Update, 35*(10), 1,4–6.

Zaragoza, N., Vaughn, S., & McIntosh, R. (1991). Social skills interventions and children with behavior problems: A review. *Behavioral Disorders, 16,* 260–275.

Zins, J. E., & Elias, M. J. (Eds.) (1993). *Promoting student success through group interventions.* New York: Haworth Press.

Index

♦

LIBRARY
ST. LOUIS COMMUNITY COLLEGE
AT FLORISSANT VALLEY.